Evaluat... ...cation
for C... ...Palsy

Philli... ...ne Hur

London : HMSO

ISBN 0 11 701716 7

Table of Contents

Acknowledgements

The DES appointed Steering Committee gave valued support and guidance during all phases of this project. Mr. Chris Dee of the DES was especially helpful during the most difficult stages of the project, and Professor Lea Pearson was also helpful at all stages of the work.

Mr. Andrew Sutton, The Birmingham Foundation for Conductive Education and the Birmingham Institute for Conductive Education allowed the evaluation to take place and we are grateful for their assistance.

Staff of the András Pető Institute for Motor Disorders, especially Julia Horvath, Ildiko Kozma and Aniko Salga, had crucial roles in the selection of the comparison group, provided the research team with much valuable information on conductive education and the workings of the Pető and Birmingham Institutes, and facilitated the assessment of children in the Birmingham Institute.

Staff of Foxdenton School, Mere Oaks School and Pictor School in Greater Manchester were invariably welcoming and helpful to the research team during the difficult process of selecting and assessing children in the comparison group.

Staff of Abbey Roman Catholic School, Ardenhurst School, Finham School, Horton Lodge School, St. Mary's School, St. Judes School and Victoria School were also welcoming and helpful to the research team during the continued assessments of children in the Birmingham and Manchester groups.

Children in the Birmingham and Manchester groups, together with parents of these children, cooperated during lengthy and demanding assessments, and their crucial role in the project is especially acknowledged.

Ms. Helen Jones had a central role in the project as clerical officer, most importantly in timetabling the assessments, assisting with the assessment of individual children, gathering background data on the children, organising travel and accommodation in the United Kingdom and abroad for various members of the research team, as well as preparing all the working papers and the final report.

Ms. Cathie Green, Research Associate, also had a vital role in the project, most importantly in checking the full data-set, compiling and managing the database, carrying out most of the statistical analyses and preparing all the figures for the final report.

Ms. Dianne Dennis was instrumental in compiling the tests making up the Language Assessment and carried out all the relevant assessments.

Ms. Jeanne Downton worked in designing the assessment of out-of-school factors possibly affecting the childrens' functioning, carried out all the relevant interviews with parents, provided valuable insights which helped in the drafting of the final report, and assisted with editing the full final draft.

Dr. John Patrick, Ms. Michelle Moore and other staff of the Orthotic Research and Locomotor Assessment Unit, Robert Jones and Agnes Hunt Orthopaedic Hospital, Oswestry, took part in the Gross-Motor Assessment and the Physical Assessment of all the children in the Birmingham and Manchester groups and their work on the project is gratefully acknowledged.

Ms. Linda Chavasse and Dr. Ilene Rusk provided assistance during the selection of the comparison children and assisted with the initial analysis of some of the data. Dr. Rusk also gathered demographic data relevant to the incidence of cerebral palsy.

Professor Judith Laszlo provided comments on drafts of the final report and her valuable contribution to the work is gratefully acknowledged.

Mr. Mark Manning and Ms. Kim Sainsbury assisted in carrying out the principal-components analysis and Ms. Sainsbury also assisted in the preparation of initial drafts of some sections of the final report.

Mr. Mervyn Bairstow willingly gave time to proof-reading and editing various drafts of various sections of the final report.

Finally, we gratefully acknowledge the co-operation and helpfulness of staff, pupils and parents of the following schools, and staff in local Health and Education Authorities during early stages of the search for comparison children: Clatterbridge (Wirral), Harold Magnay (Liverpool), Springfield (Knowsley), especially Mr. Terry Swales; and staff, patients and parents of the Child Development Centre, St. Luke's Hospital (Bradford), especially Mr. Peter Corry. Ms. Hilary Came and other staff of Richard Cloudesley School helped when parts of the research methodology were being piloted.

To all the above we give our heartfelt thanks.

Summary

Conductive education for children with cerebral palsy was imported from the András Pető Institute for Motor Disorders in Budapest to the Birmingham Institute for Conductive Education and was evaluated by a team from the School of Psychology, University of Birmingham, sponsored by the Department of Education and Science.

The first objective of the evaluation was to determine the extent to which the form of conductive education developed in Birmingham was an accurate replica of that established at the Pető Institute. Observations of programmes in Birmingham and programmes in Budapest did not reveal major differences. On the other hand, circumstances surrounding the establishment of the Birmingham Institute introduced difficulties which affected the delivery of the programmes; namely, staff were recruited and trained in a way that impaired the rapid learning of the attitudes and methods required by conductive education, children and their parents were not sufficiently prepared for conductive education, and the Birmingham Institute was relatively isolated from other educational and medical establishments relevant to the children's current and future needs. However, there is no evidence that any of these difficulties affected the children's progress.

The second objective was to make explicit the principles upon which conductive education operates, and generate hypotheses as to which of those principles may be crucial to its effective implementation. The first step of establishing the immediate objectives of conductive education was facilitated by staff from the Pető Institute. Subsequent steps of describing the long term objectives, methods and principles, had to rely on readings of English translations of Hungarian texts. The extent to which a clear and coherent account could be made was more a function of careful choice and juxtaposition of quotations than of the clarity and coherence of the texts. Proponents of conductive education should be challenged to provide a clear and comprehensive account of the system in English, which is the language understood by the majority of the world's scientific community, as a first step in having the system widely accepted. It proved impossible to identify which of the implied principles of conductive education might be crucial to its effective implementation.

The third objective was to evaluate the effectiveness of conductive education for children with cerebral palsy in the Birmingham Institute, compared to the effectiveness of some alternative British programmes. Children enrolled in schools providing special education in Greater

Manchester were identified, matched as a group in their background and on a range of abilities to those receiving conductive education in Birmingham. Progress of all children enrolled in the Institute was compared to progress of the small subset of children enrolled in the schools in Greater Manchester on a battery of tests of cognition, academic achievement, communication, motor functioning, social behaviour, independence in activities of daily living, physical state of the hips and the hamstring muscles, and neurological status. This provided a test of the effectiveness of conductive education against a standard provided by programmes in Greater Manchester but did not provide a general test of the effectiveness of those programmes because findings would not be relevant to the larger number of children enrolled in the Greater Manchester schools.

While children receiving conductive education made progress on a wide range of functional and physical measures, there was no evidence to support predictions that they would achieve better rates of progress than children receiving British programmes of special education. On the contrary, despite the fact that conditions favoured the group receiving conductive education, the only evidence for differences in their rate of development was in favour of the group in Greater Manchester. An investigation of the progress of individual children showed that while it might be possible to argue that conductive education had been a 'success' for some children it could be argued, equally, that it had been a 'failure' for others. Until it can be demonstrated that conductive education meets the expectations of its protagonists, the following conclusions are appropriate: staff involved with United Kingdom special education should be circumspect in their view of conductive education and should not feel compelled to adopt the methods which are advocated; parents of children with cerebral palsy should regard with caution the promises made on behalf of conductive education and they should not feel they are failing if they do not secure conductive education for their child.

The fourth objective was to begin to define the range of applicability of conductive education in Britain. Since systems of special education are commonly applied in the absence of proof of their effectiveness, and the Pető and Birmingham Institutes would not be unique among providers of education if they continued to offer conductive education regardless of the outcome of an evaluation, the approach taken was to consider the applicability of conductive education regardless of the findings about its effectiveness compared to United Kingdom special education. A wide range of clinical conditions and functional characteristics led to children being judged by the conductors as unsuitable for conductive education. The Pető Institute's screening procedure rejected an estimated 65 per cent of children with cerebral palsy. Pooling these children with the wide range of other childhood conditions which were not accepted, it seems that conductive education is suitable for only a minority of children with motor disorders.

Another important finding was that children at the Birmingham Institute, as a group, made only modest progress over a two year period on the conductors' own scales of development, although a small number of children showed marked improvement on some scales while there were other children who showed no improvement. The data from the conductors' assessments must be regarded as disappointing in the light of claims made on behalf of conductive education by its proponents, and do not appear to justify the widespread introduction of the system into the United Kingdom.

Background and Context

This section gives background to the present study and describes the context in which the work was carried out.

1.1   ANDRÁS PETŐ INSTITUTE FOR MOTOR DISORDERS

The András Pető Institute for Motor Disorders in Budapest is the main centre for conductive education in Hungary. The Institute's roles include maintaining a national register of motor-disordered children, training staff in the principles and practice of conductive education, and educating children and adults who fall within specific diagnostic categories (eg. cerebral palsy, spina bifida, multiple sclerosis, Parkinson's disease).

A detailed account of the development of conductive education and the history of the Pető Institute is outside the scope of the present study. Cottam and Sutton (1986) give a good introduction to the historical and social background of the Institute; "an educational system is comprehensible only when related to the wider social context of which it is a part . . . Any attempt to understand conductive education must, therefore, begin with an outline of its social-historical context" (p. 3).

Hungary embarked on a comprehensive reorganisation of existing educational provisions and the formation of a state system of education during the 1940's. The unprecedented expansion of preschool, school, and higher education was, at that time, referred to as 'the learning disease'. It could be expected that such a period would also see many innovations. Education continues to be given high priority and visitors to modern-day Hungary are often impressed by the commitment of authorities, parents and pupils to the broadest and highest possible education for all, commencing with some form of preschool education for nearly all children. A feature of Hungarian education is the emphasis on teaching music, and music also has a major role in conductive education (Sections 3.6 and 5.4.5).

Although schools for specific categories of disabilities were first established in Hungary during the 19th century, the wider provision of special education for children with disabilities dates back also to the 1940's and can be seen as part of the general expansion of education taking place at that time. Mainstream and special education, then and now, are segregated in both philosophy and practice. The basic aim of special education is to enable children who are disabled to master the curriculum and syllabus of mainstream education.

A general requirement of all mainstream and special education establishments in Hungary, relevant to an understanding of the origins and aims of conductive education, is that a child must be able to walk. Children who cannot get about satisfactorily by themselves (the use of wheelchairs is not allowed) are not permitted to attend a mainstream school or a special school and are entitled only to a limited amount of home tuition. This rule extends also to residential special schools for children with motor disabilities; children who cannot walk, cannot attend.

András Pető (1893–1967) was trained in medicine and had a special interest in rehabilitation. It was during the rapid expansion of education in the 1940's that he began to develop his system of conductive education for adults and children with motor disabilities. The process by which he developed the system and its theoretical foundation is not well recorded. There are few publications on the methods and principles of conductive education (Section 5). An early struggle for recognition, first under the Ministry of Health and later under the Ministry of Education led eventually to official acceptance in 1963. Dr. Maria Hari had helped Pető during the earliest days of the Institute and she took on his role as director soon after his death. The present Institute was formally opened in 1985. While staff from the Institute provide services elsewhere in Budapest and in a number of provincial centres, conductive education is still centralised at the Institute.

The Institute remains under the Ministry of Education but separate from the rest of special education. It has its own network of services, its own system of professional training, and is somewhat isolated even from educational and medical specialists working in closely related fields in Hungary, some of whom are staunch critics of the system. In contrast to other education establishments, the Institute accepts children with motor disorders even if they cannot walk. It does not aim to provide for the long-term educational needs of children but rather to prepare them for acceptance into a mainstream school or special school. Such acceptance depends on the children being able to get about by themselves, take part in lessons, use stairs, normal furniture, toilets etc. Criteria for discharge from the Institute and acceptance into a mainstream school or special school do not seem to be comprehensively and unambiguously documented (Section 5.3). An evaluation of the efficacy of conductive education using research methods acceptable to the scientific community has never been carried out (Sutton, 1987).

1.2 BIRMINGHAM FOUNDATION FOR CONDUCTIVE EDUCATION

The Pető Institute apparently did not instigate the current world-wide drive to establish conductive education outside Hungary. Rather, interest in conductive education (within the United Kingdom in particular) grew as a result of professionals and parents visiting the Institute in Budapest, especially from the 1960's onward (Cottam and Sutton, 1986; Cotton, 1965). Such visitors witnessed practices which seemed compellingly different from anything they knew. Programmes appeared highly structured with clear goals and both staff and children demonstrated a indefatigable involvement during long days of intense work. There were also reports of high success in getting severely disabled children to function independent of physical aids and personal assistance.

The first attempt to introduce conductive education in Britain was made in 1970 by a physiotherapist working for the Spastics Society at a special school for children with cerebral palsy, Mrs. Ester Cotton (Cotton, 1986). She spent time in Budapest, developed a system based on principles of conductive education and widely published her observations, experiences and ideas. There are now many other schools in the United Kingdom which have programmes 'based on the principles of conductive education' (eg., Corbett and Loring, 1989).

During the 1980's newspaper, radio and television news media produced accounts of conductive education and of individual children from the United Kingdom apparently benefiting greatly from periods at the Pető Institute. These accounts were widely noticed (eg., Lonton and Russell, 1989; Patrick, 1989) and stimulated a nationwide drive, largely parent led, to have conductive education, as provided at the Pető Institute, introduced for the first time into the United Kingdom.

The Foundation for Conductive Education, a national charity, was formed to meet this demand (see Pearson (1991) for a good account of the history of the Foundation and Institute for Conductive Education). Support initially came from local government, various organisations concerned with disabled children and adults, as well as companies and individuals. The Foundation negotiated an agreement with the Pető Institute to transfer conductive education, initially on a small scale, to its first sponsored project, the Birmingham Institute for Conductive Education. Beside the immediate task of promoting the work of the Institute, the Foundation promotes conductive education nation-wide, lobbies individuals and organisations for support, engages in fund raising activities, and aims to establish a National Institute for Conductive Education.

1.3 BIRMINGHAM INSTITUTE FOR CONDUCTIVE EDUCATION

It follows from the quote in Section 1.1 that the context in which a system of education develops, normally determines to some extent the nature and objectives of that system. Yet the aim of the Foundation for Conductive Education (Section 1.2), perhaps unprecedented in the United Kingdom, was to implant a system of education into a British context that was historically and socially very different to the Hungarian context that gave it birth. For example, unlike Hungary in the 1940's, systems of special education for all children with disabilities already existed in Britain. Furthermore, the criteria for acceptance into schools and the demands of society as a whole are different from those in Hungary. There was no requirement for a British institute, with a role like the Pető Institute, to prepare children for acceptance into schools. There is a tradition in Britain of structuring the environment in schools and elsewhere to take account of the needs of children and adults with disabilities, in contrast to Hungary where there is an expectation that individuals with disabilities should adapt to a normal environment. In the above light, the Foundation's objective of implanting conductive education in the United Kingdom was unusual, to say the least, and it was reasonable to suppose that there would be difficulties in the pursuit of the objective (Section 4).

The Birmingham Institute for Conductive Education opened in September 1987 with the following aims: to train British school teachers in the principles and practice of conductive education; to educate children with cerebral palsy using the methods of conductive education (later educate adults with Parkinson's disease); and to make possible a scientific evaluation of conductive education as provided at the Birmingham Institute.

The Institute was established for an initial period of four years, taking account of the fact that the training course for a conductor (the title given to a qualified practitioner of conductive education) covers four years. The Project Director appointed at the Birmingham Institute was a qualified British teacher and a support teacher was appointed later; neither were qualified as conductors. Ten qualified British school teachers were recruited as trainee conductors, although five were to withdraw before graduating. Training took place at the Birmingham Institute for half of each year, during which time the trainees were instructed and supervised by Hungarian conductors resident in Birmingham. For the rest of the year training took place at the Pető Institute. During these periods the trainees were replaced in Birmingham by qualified Hungarian conductors. There was an administrative and support staff, but until 1990 there was no medical or paramedical staff. [Later intakes of trainees received all their training in Budapest.]

Ten children with cerebral palsy were initially enrolled. They commenced their conductive education in January 1988 at the Pető Institute where the British trainee conductors were also receiving their initial training. The children and the trainees returned to Birmingham and commenced work at the Institute in September 1988. These children and an additional ten children, enrolled between this date and January 1990, were included in the present study.

The third role of the Birmingham Institute, namely to make possible a research evaluation of conductive education, was determined at the time of the Institute's creation (Sutton, 1987). Major sponsors committed funds for the provision of conductive education on the condition that the work of the Institute would be evaluated. It was not intended that the Institute would, itself, carry out the evaluation but rather the research would be funded and staffed as a separate undertaking, though integrated with other functions of the Institute.

Agreements between the Foundation for Conductive Education and the Pető Institute gave the Pető Institute the following broad roles in the Birmingham Institute: screening children with cerebral palsy for suitability for conductive education, deciding who should be enrolled and when they should be discharged; theoretical and practical training of trainee conductors in Birmingham and in Budapest and examining their progress; educating the children as closely as possible in accord with the principles of conductive education. There was, however, no firm initial agreement covering the research evaluation of the Birmingham Institute's work and this had implications for the conduct of the research.

1.4 EVALUATION OF CONDUCTIVE EDUCATION

A response of central government to the widespread publicity given to conductive education in the 1980's (Section 1.2) was to fund the evaluation of work to be carried out at the Birmingham Institute. A grant was awarded by the Department of Education and Science to the School of Psychology, University of Birmingham for research with the following objectives:

1. To determine the extent to which the form of conductive education developed in Birmingham is an accurate replica of that established at the Pető Institute.

2. To make explicit the principles upon which conductive education operates, and generate hypotheses as to which of those principles may be crucial to its effective implementation.

3. To evaluate the effectiveness of conductive education for children with cerebral palsy in the Birmingham Institute, compared to the effectiveness of some alternative British programmes.

4. To begin to define the range of applicability of conductive education in Britain.

Work commenced in July 1987 with the appointment of a Research Fellow. A Senior Research Fellow, later Research Director, was appointed in March 1988 and a clerical officer in April 1988. The Research Fellow resigned and was replaced in July 1988. Other Research Fellows and Research Associates were employed on a short term basis over the period of the study, and a half-time Research Fellow joined the project for the final year. In addition to the staff based at the School of Psychology a range of other professionals were engaged on the project, including, an orthopaedic surgeon, speech therapist, physiotherapist and a social worker.

The original research timetable allowed for a three year study of children receiving conductive education at the Birmingham Institute and of comparison children in alternative programmes of special education (Objective 3). The other three research objectives would be worked on in parallel with the longitudinal study. The final report was due in July 1992. In the meantime, the research team was required to report periodically to a Steering Committee set up by the Department of Education and Science. The team also provided information to a Local Management Committee which represented major sponsors of conductive education and oversaw the operation of the Birmingham Institue. The research project was not, however, under the control of either the Institute or the Foundation; ie., the evaluation project was funded and staffed independently of the provision of conductive education.

There was a major problem for the research in addressing Objectives 1, 2 and 4, stemming from the need for discussion and some collaborative work with staff of the Pető Institue over a three year period. Different staff, speaking with authority, often expressed different and sometimes even opposing views on key features of conductive education, and there was evidence of major changes in view over the short period of this study. The research team found this surprising because conductive education has a history exceeding forty years and gives the impression, initially at least, of being well defined even to the extent of being rigid in its specifications. Problems for the research were exacerbated by the lack of comprehensive and coherent publications on the objectives, methods and principles of conductive education (Section 5).

The team was left with the impression that after a long period of relative stability, conductive education, from the mid 1980's onward, entered a period of change. Considerable international pressure for increased availability of conductive education may have resulted in a loosening of previously rigid standards, which may be a cause of the lack of consensus among staff in their views. Changes will probably continue to occur and it is necessary, therefore, to point out that statements relating to conductive education made in the present report pertain to conditions prevailing in the Pető and Birmingham Institutes over the period of this study, and may not be accurate or relevant in the future.

Cerebral Palsy

PART II

2

2.1 INTRODUCTION

Cerebral palsy is a chronic disorder due to non-progressive damage to the brain and appears before the age of three years. It is marked primarily by faulty control of posture and movement but there can be other disabilities. It is difficult to generalise when discussing cerebral palsy because there are multiple causes and damage to the brain is highly variable, resulting in a unique pattern of disabilities in each child. The absence of universally agreed standards of assessment, diagnosis and classification (Blair and Stanley, 1985; Gans and Glenn, 1990) complicates any attempt to review relevant literature.

2.2 INCIDENCE AND AETIOLOGY

The early diagnosis of cerebral palsy is often difficult and the lack of consistency in criteria employed, may partly explain the wide variation in reported incidence from two to five per 1000 live births (Evans et al, 1985). The incidence may not have changed much in recent years (Hagberg, Hagberg and Zetterstrom, 1989; Rang and Wright, 1989; Stanley, 1987) because, while it has been possible to eliminate some causes, advanced medical care of premature babies has increased their survival rate and 'prematurity' is one of the predisposing factors (Shields and Schifrin, 1988; Stanley and English, 1986; Torfs et al, 1990).

Children with cerebral palsy are found in all types of families regardless of nationality, race or socioeconomic grouping. More boys than girls are affected but genetic abnormalities are uncommon and there is often no history of other cases in the family. The disorder usually originates before or during birth and most cases are, therefore, 'congenital' although problems may not be apparent at birth. After a variable period it can be the mother who first notices something odd: there might be a feeding problem, with the infant not sucking well or swallowing well; there may be unusual stiffness in the arms or legs, or overall excessive floppiness; the infant may show constant irritability, may sleep poorly, or may show no reaction to sudden movement or loud noises. A diagnosis is often made only after many examinations, but by the age of two years most congenital cases have been diagnosed.

It is often very difficult to pin-point the cause of cerebral palsy in an individual child and it is likely that most cases are brought about by a number of factors operating together (Stanley and English, 1986; Torfs et al, 1990). The recent application of computed tomography in the study of cerebral palsy (Schouman-Claeys et al, 1989; Yokochi et al, 1989) and neurophysiological studies (eg., Leonard et al, 1990; Whitlock, 1990) may assist in understanding the aetiology of the disorder. Possible causes can be grouped as follows.

Prenatal. Events between the time of conception and the onset of labour can interfere with the development of the brain; eg., problems with the placenta, infections suffered by the mother like rubella or viral infections, metabolic diseases in the mother like diabetes or hyperthyroidism, mother's medication, alcohol or drug abuse.

Perinatal. A range of events occurring between the onset of labour and actual birth can cause brain damage leading to cerebral palsy; eg., obstruction of the umbilical cord or later obstruction of the respiratory pathway both resulting in lack of oxygen, injury to the head during labour causing haemorrhage in the brain, delivery that is too rapid or too slow resulting in excessive pressure changes to the head and interference with blood supply, prematurity with birth occurring before the brain is sufficiently developed.

Postnatal. Less common than the above 'congenital' types of cerebral palsy, 'acquired' cerebral palsy can result from events occurring in the first two years of life; eg., trauma to the head, infections resulting in meningitis or encephalitis, neoplasms.

2.3 CLASSIFICATION

Cerebral palsy is classified on motor criteria according to the part of the body affected, the type of motor disability and the overall severity of the disability although there are no universally agreed standards (Evans and Alberman, 1985; Gans and Glenn, 1990; Jarvis and Hey, 1984; Phelps, 1990). The following are the most commonly occurring terms:

When only one side of the body is clearly affected the term 'right-hemiplegia' or 'left-hemiplegia' is used. 'Diplegia' is used when the lower limbs are affected more than the upper limbs, while 'quadriplegia' applies when all four limbs are involved.

A number of terms are used to describe the different types of motor disability which can be found. The 'spastic' type of cerebral palsy occurs when the motor cortex or cerebrum has been damaged. The muscles are tight, will not easily lengthen when the limbs are passively manipulated and the child's own movements appear jerky and poorly controlled. When basal parts of the brain have been damaged, the term 'athetoid' is applied to indicate the slow, irregular, twisting and uncoordinated movements which occur whenever the child attempts to carry out an action. Problems with balance caused by damage to the cerebellum are indicated by the use of the term 'ataxic'.

Children with cerebral palsy vary greatly in the severity of their motor difficulties. There is no standardized scale of motor disability but the terms 'mild', 'moderate', and 'severe' are frequently applied as indications of the overall magnitude of the motor problems.

2.4   ASSOCIATED PROBLEMS

Most children with cerebral palsy have other difficulties (Evans et al, 1985) in addition to motor problems in the limbs and trunk. The pattern and severity of difficulties depends on the extent, site and timing of damage to the brain, as well as the effects of any remediation such as medical or surgical intervention.

Other motor problems. Parts of the brain controlling muscles concerned with eye movement (Mayberry and Gilligan, 1985), swallowing and the speech apparatus can be impaired, leading to problems with vision, feeding and verbal communication.

Orthopaedic problems. Contractures (Bax and Brown, 1985) in various muscle groups can lead to distorted postures involving the wrist, elbow, hips, knees or ankles. Prolonged or severe contractures can result in dislocation of the hip (Cooke, Cole and Carey, 1989), for example, as well as a variety of fixed deformities because muscle growth is affected by muscle stretching and bone growth is affected by the pull exerted by the muscles.

Cognitive dysfunction. Many children with cerebral palsy have some form of cognitive dysfunction (Banich et al, 1990; Lesny et al, 1990; Parette and Hourcade, 1984), the severity of which does not necessarily match the severity of the motor difficulties (McCarty et al, 1986). For example, some children with mild cerebral palsy, function poorly on tests of general mental ability. On the other hand, despite considerable difficulties in assessing the cognitive functioning of children with severe motor and speech problems, there are some children who manage to demonstrate superior abilities on intelligence tests.

Communication disorders. Many children with cerebral palsy have problems with communication which can stem from a variety of causes. Some children have a partial or complete hearing loss which interferes with their reception of speech. Others have normal hearing but fail to understand speech due to a problem in the central processing of auditory input. Disorders of the speech apparatus, such as problems with control of the tongue, lips, palate or breathing, can result in partial or complete inability to make speech sounds. Other children have adequate control of the speech apparatus but fail to use it for verbal expression, due to central problems with the use of language. Some children who have problems with verbal expression also have problems with non-verbal expression, because general difficulties in motor control can prevent the use of the hands, and of facial expressions, for communication.

Visual and other perceptual dysfunctions.　Most visual problems (eg., Wedell, 1960) in children with cerebral palsy are caused by disorders in control over muscles of the eye. For example, difficulties with the visual fixation of stationary and moving objects interfere with the formation of a stable retinal image essential for good vision, while problems with convergence and focusing of the eyes interfere with stereopsis. Other perceptual problems reported in cerebral palsy involve the tactile and kinaesthetic systems (Bolanos et al, 1989; Lee, Turnbull and Cook, 1989).

Seizures.　The majority of children with cerebral palsy experience seizures at some stage during their development. Seizures can cause many secondary social and behavioural problems in addition to major disruptions to learning and performance. Drugs which may be administered to control seizures can have secondary effects including the impairment of function.

Behavioural and social problems.　A variety of behavioural problems can be apparent; eg., short attention span, impulsive behaviour, distractability, hyperactivity. Such behaviour can be disruptive in a group situation and can interefere with therapy programmes, education programmes and the development of interpersonal relationships. Even without such behavioural problems, however, children with motor and communication problems can be impaired in their interpersonal development because of reduced opportunity to interact with other children and adults, for example. Furthermore, on reaching adulthood, individuals can experience problems with self-esteem (Magill-Evans and Restall, 1991).

Other problems

A range of factors including problems with muscle growth (O'Dwyer, Neilson and Nash, 1989), loss of power and fatiguability in the upper limb (Brown et al, 1987), abnormal energy expenditure during gross-motor activities (Fernandez, Pitetti and Betzen, 1990; Rose et al, 1990) can contribute to difficulties in achieving independence in activities of daily living (Bleck, 1990).

2.5　MANAGEMENT

There is no 'cure' for cerebral palsy (Gans and Glen, 1990) and while the underlying neurological problem is not progressive there may be compensatory re-organisation in central pathways (Farmer et al, 1991), and there can be a gradual change in the manifestations of the disorder (Nelson and Ellenberg, 1982). Neurological signs (Watt, Robertson and Grace, 1989) change during the first few years as the central nervous system matures, and functional compensations can proceed over a much longer time course. On the other hand, chronic imbalance in the action of muscle groups can lead to progressive physical deformity, while increase in the size of the body especially at puberty can be accompanied by loss of previously acquired abilities to control posture and mobility.

There is a generally prevailing view that most children with cerebral palsy can be helped to improve their functioning. Intervention broadly aims to maximise function in the area of a disability or else to provide a means by which a difficulty can be by-passed. Orthopaedic surgery involving the tendons, bones or joints can be an option in spasticity, to prevent the development of physical deformity and to improve function (Craig and Zimbler, 1990; Larsson et al, 1986), while selective dorsal rhizotomy has also been used to counter spasticity (Abbott, Forem and Johann, 1989; Peacock and Staudt, 1991; Vaughan, Berman and Peacock, 1991). Drugs acting centrally and peripherally can be used to reduce spasticity and drug therapy is also used extensively to control seizures (Glen, 1990; Whyte and Robinson, 1990). Plaster casting (Hinderer et al, 1988; Walsh et al, 1990), orthotic devices such as splints (Feldman, 1990; Hylton, 1990; Tardieu et al, 1988) and infant walkers (Holm, Harthun-Smith and Tada, 1983) have been used to stretch muscles, improve upper limb function and mobility. Special seating and other devices for positioning can improve posture and provide support for optimal head control and hand function, for example (Hallenborg, 1990; McPherson et al, 1991; Myhr and Von Wendt, 1991). Physiotherapy, occupational therapy, speech therapy, augmentative communication aids, biofeedback, relaxation, behaviour modification, and the use of heat, cold, vibration and massage are all used in various contexts with the aim of controlling spasticity, preventing contractures and improving posture, mobility, hand function, communication and independence in activities of daily living (Bax, 1986; Bax and Brown, 1985; Bourget, McArtor and Roolstown, 1989; Diamond, 1986; Giebler, 1990; Hill, 1985; Kanda et al, 1984; Karlsson, Nauman and Gardestrom, 1960; Laskas et al, 1985; Nash, Neilson and O'Dwyer, 1989; O'Donoghue, 1988; Palmer et al, 1988; Parette, Holder and Sears, 1984; Parette and Hourcade, 1984; Sparling, 1988; Udwin and Yule, 1990; Whyte and Morrissey, 1990). Evidence for the effectiveness of various forms of intervention is patchy (Rang and Wright, 1989) but one important predictor of whether children will benefit may be general cognitive ability, with children of higher ability benefitting most (Banich et al, 1990; Goldkamp, 1984; Karlsson, Nauman and Gardestrom, 1960; Parette and Hourcade, 1984). Finally, some children can cope with the demands of a full mainstream school programme which will prepare them for maximum independence, employment or higher education.

Family counselling and support as early as possible (Diamond, 1986) is crucial to the management of the children. Parents often need specialist information and help in the early years if they are to come to terms with having a child who has a variety of difficulties and to learn about the network of specialist services which are potentially available for treatment, management and education. Parents also need guidance on how best to manage the child at home. There can be difficulties in the interaction between parent and child (Hanzlik, 1990; Rosenberg and Robinson, 1988) yet the parent can have an important role in promoting the child's development (Robinson, Rosenberg and Beckman, 1988). Siblings can be instructed about cerebral palsy and this can also help development (Craft et al, 1990).

There is reduced life expectancy among individuals with cerebral palsy (Evans and Alberman, 1990) and most remain dependent, in one way or another, on help from the family or from professional services. On the other hand, many achieve complete independence in activities of daily living, earn a living in sheltered or even non-sheltered circumstances and marry and have children. The aim of anyone concerned with the problems of cerebral palsy must be to provide conditions which enable an individual to make use of existing abilities, to overcome difficulties and to fulfil potential as far as possible.

Conductive Education and United Kingdom Special Education

3.1   INTRODUCTION

The main subject of this report is an evaluation of conductive education as provided at the Birmingham Institute. Objective 3 (Section 1.4) required a study of the effectiveness of conductive education for children with cerebral palsy compared to the effectiveness of some alternative British programmes. It was necessary, therefore, to follow the development of the group of children in the Birmingham Institute but also to identify and follow a comparison group of children enrolled in traditional programmes. This requires a description of conductive education and United Kingdom special education.

Given that a major thrust of the study is a comparison between contrasting forms of special education in their efficacy, the features which seem to illustrate the contrasts most clearly will be singled out for discussion. A comprehensive account of each of the programmes will not be attempted.

The programme at the Birmingham Institute should have been the source of information about conductive education for the present section. However, since the programme was being established during the period of this study, the present account will be based on the provision at the Pető Institute which was the model being copied in Birmingham. This section will be followed with an account of whether conductive education as practised in Birmingham at the time of this study was an accurate replica of that provided at the Pető Institute (Section 4), thus fulfilling Objective 1 (Section 1.4).

There is no 'national system' of special education for children with cerebral palsy in the United Kingdom, and there are variations between schools including the three schools in Greater Manchester from which the comparison group was drawn (Section 6.4). For example, it became clear through observations and discussions that the three schools differed with respect to the extent of collaboration with parents for ensuring continuity between educational practices at school and practices at home, and the schools had different methods for transferring children into alternative educational settings (the issue of 'continuity' Section 3.3). The schools also differed on matters relating to the 'programme' (Section 3.6); eg., in one school, therapists carried out a lot of work in the class setting, while in the other two schools, children tended to be withdrawn from the class for individualised programmes. On the other hand, programmes in the different schools have much in common and differences between them are far smaller than obvious contrasts between United Kingdom programmes and conductive education. The present account of United Kingdom special education, therefore, is an 'amalgam' based on the three schools which, in turn, have much in common with schools elsewhere in the United Kingdom.

Information on conductive education and United Kingdom special education was gathered during periods of direct observation of the programmes in Budapest and Manchester, supplemented by discussions held with staff involved with the delivery of the programmes. Accounts of conductive education originating from the Pető Institute, can be found in Hari and Akos (1988) and Hari and Tillemans (1984) while there are several other accounts published by professionals not employed by the Pető Institute (eg., Cottam and Sutton, 1986; Jernqvist, 1986; Presland, 1991). Further details regarding conductive education can be found in Section 5 of the present report.

3.2   CLASSES

Conductive education is carried out with specifically composed groups (Section 5.4.3) and there is considerable control over the type of child that is enrolled. Groups are typically homogeneous in as much as all the children are diagosed cerebral palsied for example, albeit they vary in the type of cerebral palsy and the severity of disability. There must be a mixture of functional abilities, and newly enrolled children are placed in existing groups, so that they can learn from those already experienced in conductive education. To maximise progress, groups are continually restructured depending on the needs of individual children and on the rate of progress of the group as a whole.

Schools providing special education in the United Kingdom are often required by external authorities to enrol children with many different types of disabilities after a minimum amount of screening. The composition of a class may largely depend on the type of child that must be enrolled from the school's catchment area. By force of circumstance, classes are often made up of children of wide ranging diagnoses (cerebral palsy, spina bifida, muscular dystrophy, rarer types of neurological disorders) and therefore a very wide range of functional abilities (HM Inspectors Report, 1989). Classes tend to be arranged according to the age of the children. Children move up to the next class at the beginning of an academic year and the class tends to remain fixed. Children in a class often do not work as a group, so the mixture of children is not particularly important.

3.3   CONTINUITY

Conductive education aims to have a continuous effect on a child's development from the earliest contact. Children who can be brought to the Pető Institute regularly commence at around two years of age or earlier, on a part-time basis, in a 'mother-and-baby' group. The mother has the opportunity to compare the child with others in the group, not just with 'normal' children and so is better able to judge progress. Both mother and child become acquainted with the aims and methods of conductive education and a start is made on promoting the development of activities of daily living. Continuity between practice in the Institute and practice at home is judged to be fundamentally important and is aided by having the parents attend a 'school for parents' where the importance of establishing good interaction between adult and child is emphasised. It is considered ideal for a child eventually to become a resident of the Institute, and by the time of enrolment in kindergarten at three to six years of age, a child has usually been exposed to conductive education already. A child may continue on with schooling at the Institute. Whenever a child is to be discharged into a mainstream or special school, at kindergarten or school age, it is considered desirable that the child be prepared for the transition and desirable for there to be a period of aftercare during which staff from the Institute have an advisory role in promoting the principles of conductive education in the context of the next programme.

United Kingdom special education typically does not have the emphasis on continuity of educational practice from the earliest age, or continuity between practice at school and practice at home, as seen in conductive education. Detailed educational and medical reports may accompany a child when moving between educational establishments but the child may move between systems with different aims and methods, having had little preparation for the transition. Continuity between practice at school and practice at home has the status of being desirable rather than fundamentally important, hence the demands made on a child may vary depending on the environment.

3.4 PRACTITIONERS

Conductive education is carried out by 'conductors' only (Section 5.4.4). There is no parallel profession in the United Kingdom. School leavers, obviously with no prior professional qualifications, are recruited by a selective process in which academic record, health, personality, the ability to observe and the ability to establish contact with children are important. There is a unique system of in-service training with trainees engaged in delivering conductive education to children from the first year while also receiving formal tuition. Conductors are responsible for all aspects of a child's education and development, and most aspects of everyday care. In addition to school work, they are responsible for teaching the children to improve their posture, mobility and hand function, and the use of motor abilities to perform activities of daily living like feeding and dressing. They are responsible for improving the ability to communicate mainly verbally, and for the promotion of personal and interpersonal social skills. Finally, the conductors perform nursing functions like helping with bathing and toileting and they are surrogate parents for residential pupils. From the beginning to the end of the Institute's day (getting up to going to sleep in the case of residential pupils), children are under the constant care of, and education by, conductors. Conductors often work as a team with one leading the programme, others facilitating the actions of individual children while others make preparations for the next part of the programme to avoid gaps. The grouping of conductors is considered as important for successful practice as the grouping of children and it is important that conductors do not become 'attached' to individual children.

United Kingdom special education is typically staffed by several different types of professionals, recruited primarily according to academic record, trained in different traditions and employed by different authorities. Responsibility for a child's education, development and everyday care is divided between school teachers, occupational therapists, physiotherapists, speech therapists, nurses and classroom assistants, with school teachers having, perhaps, the major role. Different professionals tend to work as individuals and the level of coordination among them is below that which is seen in a group of conductors. Staff tend to become 'attached' to individual pupils during the school year because they are responsible for individuals.

3.5 AIMS

Conductive education aims to promote a broad spectrum of development in cognitive, communication, motor, social and daily living skills (Section 5.2). All areas are equally important. Children are challenged to find a way of dealing with their problems with minimum recourse to physical aids or personal assistance, to prepare them for acceptance into a mainstream or special school (Section 1.1) and, ultimately, for participation in society as fully and as independently as possible, with minimum adaptation of the social and physical environment. This latter state of function is, perhaps, what is meant by the much quoted term, 'orthofunction'. There seems to be no absolute standard for orthofunction which all children should reach. Rather, some readings seem to suggest it is a state in which an individual child has fully realized all potentials and is functioning within a minimally adapted environment (Section 5.3).

The main route to this state of independent functioning involves encouraging the children, through specifically designed programmes, to overcome their motor difficulties and be independent in posture, mobility and hand function. This demands a singular absence of special aids. For example, children are challenged to walk, to use ordinary pen and paper, and to communicate through speech only. But conductive education is not just about the promotion of motor function. The claim is that the short-term aim of strongly promoting independent motor functioning has widespread secondary benefits, eg., encouragement of problem solving attitudes and achievement motivation, important for learning in general; encouragement of independence in activities of daily living which, in turn, promotes normal social interactions and development of interpersonal relationships.

United Kingdom special education also aims to promote a broad spectrum of development in cognitive, communication, motor, social and daily living skills. However, while there is an intention to prepare children to participate in society as fully as possible, there is no requirement to restrict adaptations to the environment. This allows for different short-term aims and more varied methods of promoting development than in conductive education. There is no requirement always to promote function independent of physical aids. Indeed, it would be considered perverse to deny a child with a severe motor disorder the use of a physical aid to facilitate finding a way round the disorder for the achievement of a non-motor goal. Proving ways round severe difficulties and enabling a child to achieve as much as possible by the easiest means, is a route to the encouragement of problem solving attitudes and achievement motivation which is different from conductive education.

3.6 PROGRAMMES

Once children are of school age, conductive education requires long days of intense work; 08.00 hrs to 17.00 hrs for non-residents, 07.00 hrs to 20.00 hrs for residents. The physical environment in which the children work appears 'spartan' and is notable for the lack of specialised equipment because it is a fundamental principle of conductive education that the layout, furniture and fittings should be as normal as possible. There are, however, certain key features in the environment; namely, multi-purpose ladder-backed chairs used for sitting, standing and walking programmes and for school work; multi-purpose slatted plinths used for lying, sitting and standing programmes, and as beds and tables. There are sticks and bars for walking, slatted stools, footrests, splints and modified footwear. Even this limited range of unsophisticated apparatus is not, however, given as a means of avoiding difficult motor functions, but rather as a means of facilitating actions while attempts are made to overcome the difficulties.

Conductors facilitate the actions of children (Section 5.4.6) by having good contact with the children, by providing verbal instruction, verbal encouragement and immediate praise when difficulties are overcome, but give only minimum physical assistance, if needed, to keep a child progressing with a task. Children are made to realise that everything comes from their own efforts. There is an understanding that hard work is required from everyone although no-one will be forced beyond their abilities.

All conductive education is carried out in groups (Section 5.4.3) and it is rare for a child to be withdrawn for an individual programme. There is often a striking appearance of uniformity of action (Section 6.7.3.3) as children work at the one task like a coordinated team, although the precise purpose of the activity may vary from child to child. Each child is made to feel responsible to the group—a responsibility to 'keep up' with everyone else—and is therefore not inclined to be disruptive. The group reciprocates by providing verbal and emotional support to the individual. All this is meant to facilitate the performance of the given task but also to promote social development.

Programmes are highly structured and generally commence with a pleasant activity like singing, aimed at gaining the group's attention and cooperation. Each part of a programme may then be introduced with a clear statement of the goal. The goal might be said or sung by the group as a whole and the action carried out as the group counts, recites or sings aloud (Section 5.4.5). Verbalising the intention and then counting or singing during the action, helps to focus the child's attention on the immediate task to the exclusion of possible distractions. A programme often has a concluding section in which a conductor may review the work which has been carried out and praise the progress of individual children.

The day is clearly divided up into different periods with most time being spent on movement education in sitting programmes, walking programmes, etc, (task series, Section 5.4.2.2) and on the promotion of independence in activities of daily living like dressing, feeding and toileting (the daily schedule, Section 5.4.2.1). There is also a school programme which focuses on handwriting, arithmetic and reading with other subjects being incorporated at more advanced stages (Section 5.4.2.3). The school programme is not considered separate from the rest of conductive education and there are links to 'task series'; for example, a hand writing programme will be prefaced by a brief recapitulation of earlier sitting and finger movement programmes. There is very little 'unstructured' time or time away from supervision by conductors (Section 5.4.2.4) when children can feel free to pursue activities of their own choice by what ever means they wish.

United Kingdom special education often involves shorter days of work; perhaps 09.00 hrs to 15.30 hrs. The physical environment is quite different from that of conductive education and appears enriched by comparison. It often includes many special features in layout, furniture and fittings; for example, as far as possible all areas are on one level and if this is not the case, ramps and lifts are provided rather than just stairs. There can be a plethora of specialised and often custom-made furniture and aids which have two categories of function. First, like conductive education, there are aids which provide a means of facilitating actions during attempts to perform motor functions; eg., splints, sticks and rollators to facilitate walking. But second, unlike conductive education, there are aids which enable a child to avoid difficult motor functions in particular situations; eg. wheelchairs when quick mobility is required, special seats giving maximum support when optimal hand function is required, communication aids giving non-verbal means of expression when it is necessary for a non-speaking child to communicate. Besides the many special features, there can also be a range of situations which give the child experience at functioning in an everyday environment; for example, a library, a kitchen to prepare food, simulated bedrooms and shops for the practice of life skills. A swimming pool is also a common feature which can be used for exercises of a recreational and enjoyable nature.

Children come into contact with a range of staff who will give help, verbally and physically, when difficulties are encountered. Children generally expect assistance from others and come to understand that their environment will provide help if needed in particular circumstances.

Education is not always a group activity (Section 6.7.3.3). A class in action can have a fragmented appearance with children doing different things at the one time. There is a lot of one-to-one teaching even in the class situation and it is common for a child to be withdrawn from class for an individual programme.

Programmes generally do not have the highly structured appearance of those seen in conductive education perhaps because the classes are more heterogeneous, more individualised goals have been set and there is not much scope for large scale coordination of activities.

The day is divided up into different periods but less time is spent on movement education than is the case in conductive education (Section 6.7.3.3) and programmes in different periods tend to be independent of one another. However, specialists involved in the delivery of an individual-ised programme do, sometimes, attend other classes to encourage general-isation in the expression of a skill; eg., a therapist may attend an academic programme to encourage a better sitting posture or better hand function. The provision of 'unstructured' time in which the children can feel free to pursue activities of their own choice, using their own favoured means of mobility or expression, is considered to be beneficial for the child in, for example, promoting social development.

3.7 POSSIBLE DIFFERENCES IN THE EFFECTIVENESS OF CONDUCTIVE EDUCATION AND UNITED KINGDOM SPECIAL EDUCATION (OBJECTIVE 3)

While there have been reports of conductive education being highly successful in achieving its goals, it is very difficult to assess their validity. The reports are largely based on the library of case histories accumulated on children who have passed through the Institute. However, only children who are predicted to benefit are selected at the outset, yet the criteria for selection are not documented and the methods used for measuring progress are not standardized. Furthermore, there is no documentation of the childrens' development over a period prior to their enrolment and it would, therefore, be difficult to identify any effect of conductive education from the case histories. Indeed, a single-subject type of design for evaluating success would be impossible to implement given the method of gradual induction of children (Section 3.3). A group comparison design for evaluating success would have been possible at least in theory, but there is no record of a matched group of children enrolled in an alternative programme ever having been studied (Sutton, 1987).

On the other hand, the overall efficacy of United Kingdom special education, or of components such as therapy programmes, have not been studied in ways that would allow a ready comparison with the claims made for conductive education. Indeed, evidence that methods of intervention like those employed in the United Kingdom result in better development than that which occurs spontaneously is, at best, equivocal (Goldkamp, 1984; Kanda et al., 1984; Karlsson, Nauman and Gardestrom, 1960; Nelson and Ellenberg, 1982; Palmer et al., 1988; Parette and Hourcade, 1984; Rang and Wright, 1989).

Given that there are no existing data on which to base predictions on the relative efficacy of the two systems of education, predictions of how two matched groups of children might develop can only be based on two considerations; first the contrasts between the systems as outlined in Sections 3.2, 3.3, 3.4, 3.5 and 3.6, second, claims for conductive education made by proponents of the system.

Prediction 1.   The Foundation and Institute have a general expectation that their children will do markedly better than those in United Kingdom programmes—this is the belief that underpins the considerable effort spent on importing conductive education. Conductive education certainly places greater emphasis on improving motor function (Section 5.4) with a larger proportion of the day being spent on motor programmes of various kinds (Section 6.7.3.3). Conductive education also claims to place greater importance on promoting social abilities needed for good interpersonal relationships because close interaction and good social contact between conductors and children is the key to good practice (Section 5.4). On the other hand, United Kingdom special education seems to allow greater scope for the development of cognitive, academic (Section 6.7.3.3) and communication skills because children are provided with various means of avoiding difficult motor actions when pursuing non-motor goals in the school curriculum and in acquiring non-verbal means of communication. Practitioners of conductive education, however, claim that their pro-grammes aim to affect all domains of function simultaneously and all aspects of development are emphasised equally; this is fostered by having only one type of professional delivering the programme. Conductive education seems to provide programmes which are more intensive, with fewer gaps, less unstructured time, and with greater continuity than United Kingdom special education. It is hypothesised, therefore, that conductive education will result in better development of cognitive, communication, motor, social and daily living skills than United Kingdom special education. The high degree of selection and the specific grouping of children for conductive education should foster optimal development within the system, while United Kingdom special education must cope with imposed groupings of children which may not be ideal for progress.

Prediction 2. Children receiving conductive education are always educated in a group; they work simultaneously at a given task like a coordinated team and are therefore all exposed to the same programme. Children in United Kingdom special education are often taught on a one-to-one basis and receive many individualised programmes depending on their disabilities and potentials. It can be predicted that variance among children receiving conductive education should decrease more than variance in a group receiving United Kingdom special education.

Prediction 3. The above predictions could be verified using criterion-referenced tests of function because matched groups of children would be directly compared. The claims of conductive education, however, allow for an additional test of efficacy. Some definitions of orthofunction seem to imply that conductive education aims to normalise function (Section 5.3); ie., to get children to function to the maximum of their potential within a minimally adapted social and physical environment. "Conductive Education sets the same everyday goals and requirements for handicapped as for non-handicapped individuals according to age" (Hari and Akos, 1988; p.223). United Kingdom special education aims to maximise function; ie., to get children to function as well as possible but not to the exclusion of personal and physical assistance. This difference in emphasis leads to the prediction that conductive education should result in greater progress on **norm-referenced** tests of function than United Kingdom special education. Such tests have usually been normed on non-disabled children who are assumed to function within a non-adapted social and physical environment. Children receiving conductive education should make good progress against this type of functional standard.

Some Differences Between the Birmingham Institute and Petσ Institute

Which Had the Potential to Affect the Impact of Conductive Education in Birmingham

(Objective 1)

4.1   INTRODUCTION

The aim of the Foundation for Conductive Education in importing conductive education and implanting it into a British context was unusual and difficulties were, perhaps, inevitable (Pearson, 1991 reviews some of the difficulties). Conclusions on the effectiveness of conductive education need to take account of whether the Birmingham Institute was successful in replicating the system. Accordingly, Objective 1 of the evaluation was as follows: to determine the extent to which the form of conductive education developed in Birmingham is an accurate replica of that established at the Pető Institute. Features of conductive education at the Pető Institute which illustrate how it contrasts with United Kingdom special education are reviewed in Section 3. The purpose of the present section is to identify differences between the Birmingham Institute and the Pető Institute. The extent to which the differences may affect the impact of conductive education on children enrolled in Birmingham is then considered and predictions relating to the superior effectiveness of conductive education (Section 3.7) reviewed.

The formal agreements which led to the establishment of the Birmingham Institute gave the Pető Institute a key role in determining programmes delivered in Birmingham. Indeed, a dominant role for the Pető Institute was inevitable. There were no British staff qualified in conductive education when the Birmingham Institute opened, hence the Institute was dependent on directives from the Pető Institute and dependent on staff based in Birmingham who controlled the training of British staff and the education of the children. More over, for half the school year when British trainees were in Budapest the Birmingham Institute was staffed almost entirely by qualified Hungarian conductors.

Given this dominant and largely unquestioned role of the Pető Institute, and given that the Institute had much to gain from succeeding with a replication, it would be surprising if an independent evaluation team could find cause to question the fidelity of the programmes being offered. Observations of programmes in Birmingham and programmes for Hungarian children in Budapest were carried out but did not reveal any differences which could be defined enough to prompt commentary.

Programmes for international groups at the Pető Institute, on the other hand, were observed to be at odds with programmes for Hungarian children, demonstrating that it was possible to observe differences, where they exist. Programmes for the international groups should certainly not be used to compare with Birmingham, but any further comment on the differences between programmes within the Pető Institute is outside the scope of the present study.

While programmes in Birmingham appear to have been successfully modelled on the Pető Institute, circumstances surrounding the establishment of the Birmingham Institute introduced difficulties which compromised the delivery of the programmes. The research team was made aware of the difficulties outlined in the following sections through discussions with senior staff from the Pető Institute, and in most cases the difficulties were also verified by direct observation and by information from a variety of other personnel who have knowledge of the Institutes.

4.2 INTAKE OF CHILDREN

At the time of full-time enrolment in the Pető Institute, children of three to four years of age have, ideally, been prepared for conductive education (Section 3.3). This is achieved by having children begin their association with the Institute in the second year of life on a part-time basis (mother-and-baby groups) and by encouraging a particular style of parent/child interaction in the home (school for parents). Newly enrolled full-time pupils are never put together into novice groups but are placed in already working groups where there are children who will provide a model for their emerging behaviour. This method of prepared induction is necessary because of the centrality of group work to successful practice. Conductive education is a continuous process in which groups are in a state of slow flux as children pass through on their way to discharge without major disruption to the group as a whole.

The situation in Birmingham was notably different. The Institute commenced without a history of conductive education and had an initial tenure of four years which is the period needed to train conductors. Conductor training begins with kindergarten children so the Institute did not open with a mother-and-baby group but with a group of children aged three to four years. This initial intake was not only exposed to full-time conductive education without the usual preparation, but was also put together in a novice group. The latter circumstance may have been eased somewhat by having the group commence its education at the Pető Institute. Subsequent intakes of children also had no preparation because a mother-and-baby group was still not established. The unprepared introduction of children was contrary to the principle of preserving the group from major disruptions.

4.3 STAFFING

Conductive education is practised only by conductors (Section 3.4, Section 5.4.4). They deliver programmes aimed at promoting development in all domains simultaneously, with no domain being more important than any other. This requires an ability to observe the children holistically and to keep all aspects of function in mind regardless of the particular programme being delivered. The programmes have little in common with any other system of education and it is considered an advantage that trainees have no prior professional qualifications which might interfere with the holistic observation of children. Conductors generally work in groups and the mixture of conductors is just as important for the practice of conductive education as the mixture of children. Conductors of varying seniority make up a group; they work as a team in a hierarchy which changes independent of seniority. All must be prepared to give and accept help from one another as they train and work together with the children. The grouping of conductors is as fluid as their role within a group. This prevents the formation of individual ties between conductors and between conductors and children which is important for promoting group work among the children.

The Birmingham Institute opened with ten United Kingdom trainee conductors and two qualified Hungarian conductors. This initial mixture of trainees and conductors had insufficient variation in seniority which impaired the establishment of a changeable hierarchy important for group work. The Institute aimed to be fully recognised as a school, hence it was necessary to have teachers with British qualifications on staff. Accordingly, the Project Director and the trainees were all qualified teachers (Section 1.3) with previous experience in observing children but not in the holistic way demanded by conductive education. This could have interfered with one of the principles of conductive education, ie., the simultaneous promotion of all aspects of development regardless of the precise nature of a programme. They tended to continue with their previous practice of working as individuals. This not only further impaired the establishment of a changeable hierarchy but also made it more difficult for them to give and accept help from one another, and resulted in the formation of ties between conductors and children which may have impaired group work among the children. There was little scope for variation in the grouping of conductors which could have eased this situation, because there was effectively only one group.

4.4 ACTIVITIES OF DAILY LIVING

The Pető Institute considers it desirable that children be enrolled on a residential basis but the Institute also has non-residential pupils. Conductive education covers all activities of daily living and, therefore, commences each day when residential pupils get up at 07.00 hrs. The first two hours of the day are spent on getting out of bed, toileting, bathroom activities, dressing, breakfast, preparations connected with changing the room from a residential function, and preparing for the day's programme. All those activities are planned and implemented by conductors. The non-residential children arrive and take part in a shorter period of preparation in time for the commencement of the first formal programme at 09.00 hrs. Residential and non-residential children share a common programme involving activities of daily living, task series, school programme and free time until 16.30 hrs soon after which the non-residential children depart. The residential children have a further hour of programmes concerned mainly with physical activities, dinner is at 18.00 hrs, and the time between 18.30 hrs and 20.00 hrs is spent on bathroom activities, toileting, preparing for bed, as well as television and stories. All these activities are similarly planned and implemented by conductors. The Pető Institute considers that the activities for residential children which occur before 09.00 hrs and after 16.30 hrs are part of conductive education.

The Birmingham Institute did not provide residential facilities for children. Activities of daily living which occurred before and after the formal programme at the Institute were not, therefore, supervised by conductors. There was reduced opportunity for the children to practice and acquire the necessary skills within a conductive education environment and there may have been a heightened reliance on parents to manage their children at home in accordance with conductive education principles. While parents of non-residential pupils of the Pető Institute are prepared for this function in mother-and-baby groups and the school for parents, the arrangement for instructing parents in Birmingham was less formal and perhaps less effective.

4.5   SCHOOL PROGRAMME

The Pető Institute operates under the Ministry of Education and implements a school curriculum. Student conductors are recruited without competing ideas on educational practice and are trained in the methods of conductive education and the methods of school teaching simultaneously. On graduation they are qualified as conductors and school teachers. The preschool and school programmes are integral parts of conductive education.

The Birmingham Institute also functioned as a school and there was a requirement for British school teachers to be on the staff from the beginning. This introduced problems for the conductive education programme. Two key British personnel involved in delivering the school programme were not conductors and were not being formally trained, ie., the Project Director and the Support Teacher. On the other hand the trainee conductors were school teachers before becoming students of conductive education. They had their own ideas about school teaching and found it difficult to deliver the school programme in a new context. When the Institute was staffed predominantly by Hungarian conductors, the situation persisted because the Project Director and Support Teacher were still involved in delivering the school programme and the Hungarians who were not qualified British teachers were also involved in teaching. The level of integration between conductive education and the school programme was, therefore, not the same as in the Pető Institute.

4.6 OUTSIDE EXCURSIONS

The Pető Institute claims to organise visits to outside establishments, eg., theatre, zoo, museum. The Institute has methods of transport and a network of connections with establishments willing to receive and engage groups of children with cerebral palsy. Excursions outside the Institute are supervised by conductors and are an integral part of conductive education; they are part of what may broadly be termed 'environmental studies', are important for allowing the children to have experience of a wider environment than the Institute, and facilitate the longer-term integration of the children into society as a whole.

The Birmingham Institute did not organise visits to outside establishments as frequently as the Pető Institute. The programme as a whole was more 'closed' than at the Pető Institute and the children were to some extent kept separate rather than being brought into society.

4.7 MEDICAL CONSULTATION

The Pető Institute has close links with at least parts of the medical profession. The Director is both medically qualified and a conductor. One of the Deputy Directors is a neurologist. There are other medically qualified personnel on the staff, eg., a consultant orthopaedic surgeon and a consultant paediatrician. The children are examined regularly by the Institute's doctors. If the conductors become concerned about a child, doctors are available for consultation. The nature and timing of treatment, including surgery, is decided by the doctors in consultation with the conductors. There are also staff concerned with the design and manufacture of aids such as splints although these are often of a rather basic looking nature. Nonetheless, the medical and educational needs of the children are attended to by professionals working in a team. Decisions on the treatment and education of the children are seen as the joint responsibility of the conductors and the doctors.

The Birmingham Institute had no medical or paramedical personnel on staff during most of the period of the study and not all the children had consultants who worked closely with the conductors. Indeed, there were difficulties in the relationship between the Institute and some doctors dating back to the Institute's origins. Basic looking aids provided in Budapest were also provided in Birmingham and their design and purpose would not encourage cooperation with United Kingdom specialists. Medical needs which have a bearing on the function of the children tended to be dealt with separately from educational needs. The Birmingham Institute may, therefore, have found it difficult to deal with possible conflict between medical interventions which affect function and the provision of conductive education.

4.8   GROUP TRANSFER

Children judged suitable for conductive education are not arbitrarily put together in groups at the Pető Institute. Rather, they are grouped according to their background, abilities, needs and rate of progress. Different groups have the same type of programme but they vary in the rate of overall progress, ie., there are 'quick' groups and 'slow' groups. The nature of a group is important in deciding the placement of a child, and the progress of a child is contingent on the nature of the group. If a child ceases to make progress in one or more domains of behaviour, consideration is given to whether the present placement is appropriate for the child. The child may be transferred to another group more appropriate to current needs. The existence of many different groups is important for the provision of conductive education.

There was only one group at the Birmingham Institute. When a child ceased to make progress before achieving all that was considered possible in conductive education, there was no other group to which the child could be transferred. The Institute did not retain such children because it was perceived to be bad for the child, bad for the group as a whole, and a disadvantage to children on a waiting list who were believed to have the potential to benefit from conductive education. The Birmingham Institute did not, therefore, provide conditions necessary for all children to complete their conductive education.

4.9   AFTER-CARE

When a child is discharged from the Pető Institute at the end of conductive education, there is provision for after-care. Conductors are available for visiting the establishment receiving the child, either to consult with the staff or to continue with specialised programmes. The child may also return part-time to the Institute for continued work. This after-care is possible because the Pető Institute is part of the Hungarian education system, there is a history of cooperation (albeit imperfect) between the Institute and other educational establishment, and staff of different establishments are acquainted with each other's practices.

The Birmingham Institute did not have a similar level of cooperation with other establishments concerned with the education of children with cerebral palsy. The only qualified conductors at the Birmingham Institute were Hungarian who, therefore, could not be expected to have an intimate knowledge of conditions prevailing elsewhere in England. While it would have been important for the Institute to foster links with other schools, this did not happen to the same extent as in Hungary and there was a general lack of knowledge outside the Institute about the precise conditions prevailing within it. There was a low level of contact even between the Institute and the neighbouring special school from which a number of children were recruited and to which a few children were discharged. If, at the time of discharge, a child had not finished with conductive education but was being discharged because the only available group was no longer suitable, the Institute would have required a level of cooperation with the next establishment exceeding even that enjoyed by the Pető Institute if there was to be continuity in the child's education. The lack of detailed knowledge of each other's practice between the qualified conductors at the Birmingham Institute and staff in other educational establishments interfered with the smooth transition of children into a new environment and with conductive education after-care.

4.10   SUMMARY

Differences between the Pető Institute and the Birmingham Institute discussed above, can be rephrased as conditions associated with the provision of conductive education for Hungarian children in Budapest but absent, or not well established, in Birmingham.

1. Early recruitment of children into part-time groups to prepare them for full-time conductive education.

2. Variation in seniority among conductors working in a group and a changeable hierarchy.

3. Supervision of all activities of the day by conductors within a conductive education environment.

4. Delivery of the school curriculum by conductors in accordance with conductive education principles.

5. Routine visits to a variety of establishments outside the Institute which are able to receive and engage children with cerebral palsy.

6. Consultation between medically qualified professionals and conductors when decisions are made on the nature and timing of treatment affecting function.

7. More than one conductive education group allowing for the transfer of children between groups according to their progress and needs.

8. Collaboration with other establishments concerned with the education of children with cerebral palsy, facilitating after-care.

Any system of education exists within a context which includes social and professional factors. The aims and methods reflect the nature of society and the society's aspirations for children, yet the aims and methods of conductive education are not in close accord with United Kingdom society.

The recruitment and training of personnel depends on pre-existing professional and institutional structures, yet there were no existing United Kingdom structures to support the recruitment and training of conductors. The implementation of the system must be integrated with the work of outside educational and medical establishments concerned with the management and welfare of children, yet the Birmingham Institute began in isolation from such establishments which, in turn, had little notion of the work of the Institute.

Of the eight points listed above, the separation of the school programme from the rest of conductive education (Point 4) was fundamentally unavoidable, since trained conductors who were also British school teachers did not exist.

The above difficulties were acknowledged by staff from the Pető Institute. Parents and others have mentioned further difficulties which may have affected the delivery of the programmes in Birmingham (eg., possible problems in communication between Hungarian conductors and the children) but these were not investigated.

4.11 REVIEW OF PREDICTIONS RELATING TO THE SUPERIOR EFFECTIVENESS OF CONDUCTIVE EDUCATION

The orthodox view in the field of 'programme-evaluation' is that a programme should not be evaluated before it is fully established and stable. On the other hand, it was mandatory that an evaluation should begin when the Institute opened (Section 1.3) and despite the difficulties outlined in the previous sections, a number of considerations argued against delay in carrying out this particular evaluation.

First, any system of special education should be able to tolerate some compromises in the circumstances of its delivery. The Pető Institute and Birmingham Foundation were antonomous in setting up the Birmingham Institute and were, therefore, in a position to take account of factors most crucial to conductive education. Many of the difficulties discussed above would have been predictable but evidently they were not considered detrimental because the Institute opened with promises that the children would make better progress if they were enrolled in the conductive education being offered.

Second, even after difficulties were being experienced, the Pető and Birmingham Institutes continued to promise distinct advantages to children and they encouraged parents to transfer their children to conductive education.

Third, the Pető Institute accepts children from the United Kingdom for short periods of conductive education in Budapest. The totality of educational experiences of these children is very different and involves much less conductive education than the experiences of Hungarian children at the Pető Institute or British children at the Birmingham Institute. There is, however, an expectation that brief encounters with conductive education will improve the children's development more than if they remain in their United Kingdom programmes without such contact. This indicates that large compromises indeed are thought possible in the delivery of conductive education before benefits are eliminated.

Taking all these considerations into account, there is no reason to modify the predictions relating to the superior effectiveness of conductive education outlined in Section 3.7.

Principles of Conductive Education (Objective 2)

PART II

5

5.1 INTRODUCTION

At the outset of this project, few detailed accounts of conductive education had been published and it was necessary, therefore, to describe the system and, in particular, to highlight major differences between conductive education and United Kingdom special education (Section 3) since the project entailed a comparison between the systems in outcome for children with cerebral palsy (Section 6).

It was also desirable to attempt to describe the principles of conductive education in order to increase general understanding and to help guide possible future policy. If the comparative evaluation should favour conductive education, demand for it would greatly increase, although interest in the system and demand for it might persist even in the absence of a clearly favourable outcome. The identification of the principles of conductive education might facilitate an expansion in its programmes of special education, while avoiding some of the problems encountered in the attempt to produce a duplicate of the Hungarian system in Birmingham (Section 4).

Accordingly, the second objective of the project was as follows; 'make explicit the principles upon which conductive education operates, and generate hypotheses as to which of those principles may be crucial to its effective implementation'.

It was clear from the outset that work on this objective would need the collaboration of staff from the Pető Institute. Nothing has been published which gives a clear account of the theory and principles of conductive education and it was considered unlikely that an understanding of the system could be gained from unguided observations of the work of the Pető and Birmingham Institutes. Collaboration would involve a number of steps. First, since it would be difficult to investigate the principles before knowing the aims, the establishment of scales of progress for children receiving conductive education would help elucidate the immediate aims. The second step would be to describe what the accomplishment of the immediate aims is thought to lead to in the longer term. Third, the methods employed in bringing about immediate and long-term improvements would need some description and the fourth step would be an elucidation of guiding principles, in the context of the objectives and the methods.

The first of the above steps was carried out in collaboration with the Pető Institute as planned, and the work is summarised here and also in Section 7.6. Continued collaboration was, however, not possible. Even if it had been collaboration would not have guaranteed success, since previous attempts at elucidating the operating principles of, or theory underlying, conductive education have been likened to the ". . . quest for the proverbial Holy Grail" (Pearson, 1991; p. 38). The present account of the long term aims, methods and principles of conductive education therefore had to depend heavily on what could be gleaned from the publications of staff of the Pető Institute. There are other accounts of the aims, methods and principles of conductive education published by professionals not employed by the Pető Institute but these have not been relied upon because the views expressed may not be endorsed by the Pető Institute (eg., Cooper (1986), Cottam and Sutton (1986), Cotton (1986), Jernqvist (1986), Lonton and Russell (1989), Pearson (1991), Presland (1991), Sutton (1984, 1987), Woodhill (1991)).

5.2 SCALES OF DEVELOPMENT FOR CHILDREN RECEIVING CONDUCTIVE EDUCATION

The Pető Institute has a tradition of documenting the development of children receiving conductive education. Children are directly assessed by the conductors, whose reports are supplemented by photographic records. This tradition was continued at the Birmingham Institute where Hungarian conductors ensured that the development of each child was recorded using Pető Institute methodologies. Initially this did not involve the use of formal measurement, since the Pető Institute had not previously established scales along which children should progress as they attain conductive education goals.

The first step in the investigation of possible agreement between conductor's records of children's development and research assessments of their progress (Section 7.7), involved a member of the research team working with staff from the Pető Institute while they constructed scales covering the areas of function which are the foci of conductive education. These scales will be described here and are reported in full in Appendix 5.1.

Four scales were constructed in the domain of *Social Behaviour*. 'Formal group role' is concerned with how a child behaves in a group such as a class situation; in particular, whether the child will work within a group, whether the group accepts the child, and whether the child will take a leading role in the group. 'Relationships with adults' is concerned with whether a child establishes a social relationship with only a few adults or establishes relationships with many adults generally. 'Relationships with children in play or family situation' records whether a child establishes reciprocal social relationships with only a few children in a particular situation, with many children but only of a particular age, or with many children regardless of their age. 'Initiating individual contact with other people' is concerned with how a child responds to a social advance and initiates a social advance; in particular, whether a child is generally indifferent to social advances made by others, accepts contact when approached by an adult or child, or initiates and accepts social advances.

Six scales were constructed in the domain of *Upper Limb Function*. There are three scales for the right limb and three identical scales for the left limb. 'Differentiated movements of the fingers' relates to how the fingers are moved, whether the thumb and fingers can be opposed, and whether an object can be manipulated with the hand. 'Reaching' is concerned with whether a child can only reach out with support, or reach out without support, or reach out in a variety of directions. 'Holding an object' records whether a child can only grasp an object if it is placed in the hand, can grasp and hold an object but not release it, or can grasp, hold and release a variety of objects.

Five scales were constructed in the *Self-Care* domain. 'Dressing' is concerned with putting on and taking off clothes and footwear. 'Shoe-laces' relates to tieing and untying laces, while 'buttons' is concerned with doing-up and undoing buttons. 'Feeding' covers activities such as participating in feeding, feeding with fingers, feeding with cutlery with and without a mess. 'Toileting' is concerned with indicating the need, as well as the use of potty, toilet and toilet paper.

There are four scales in the domain of *Position Changing*; 'standing up from a stool and sitting down to a stool', 'standing up from the floor and sitting down to a stool', 'standing up from the floor and sitting down to the floor', 'sitting-up from supine, sitting and lying-down to supine on the plinth', 'rolling 360° on the floor commencing from supine'.

Two scales in the domain of *Walking* were constructed; 'without aids and bare-foot' and 'with aids', the latter concerned with walking with personal assistance or with the aid of furniture or sticks.

There are two scales in the domain of *Speech and Communication*. 'Speech' is concerned with attempting to speak, pronouncing only parts of words, sentence construction and clear pronunciation of words. 'Communication' is concerned with verbal and non-verbal communication, and whether communication is appropriate for the age of the child.

Finally, there are four scales in the domain of *Cognition*. 'General knowledge' is concerned with the child's knowledge of its personal and impersonal circumstances. 'Attention' relates to whether the child can attend to a task for brief moments only, attend in small groups, or attend to a task even when distractions are present. 'Learning ability' is concerned with whether a child can learn something new only with much repetition, whether something can be learned quickly, and whether something recently learned can be used with previously learned material. 'Motivation' relates to self-motivation and whether a child will spontaneously continue to work at a task.

5.3   GENERALISATION TO LONGER TERM DEVELOPMENT AND FUNCTIONING

The longer term aim of conductive education is to bring about a state of 'orthofunction' in the pupils. Orthofunction has been defined as ". . . the ability to function as members of society, to participate in the normal social settings appropriate to their age, kindergarten, school, college or work, without need for wheelchairs, ramps, special furniture, toileting arrangements, etc" (Cottam and Sutton, 1986; p. 41). Another account of the aims of conductive education is as follows: "The object of conductive education is not to accommodate the severe dysfunctional patients in an institute, or to send them to a special school, but to accomplish a basic task to render possible a normal education, travelling in the streets, self-supporting and work. In order to bring about an equilibrium between child and environment, we do not change the environment, but the adaptation of the child's constitution" (Gari, 1968, quoted in Cottam and Sutton, 1986l p.41–42). This anticipates a sanguine future for an orthofunction child, with an expectation of general self-sufficiency in a normal environment and it is a small wonder that parents and educationalists have become very interested in a system which makes these kinds of promises.

On the basis of the above descriptions or orthofunction, it would be a reasonably straight forward task to operationalise the long-term objectives of conductive education; ie., to define standards of functioning which each child should reach and to select or design scales of measurement which would document the progress made by children towards these standards. The objectives seem to encompass a range of functional domains including cognition and academic achievement, language, fine-motor and gross-motor functioning, social behaviour and independence skills which are, indeed, the domains encompassed by the conductive education scales. The standards of functioning aimed for seem to be normal standards (see Prediction 3, Section 3.7) and it would not be difficult to find published norm-referenced scales of measurement which would define the levels of functioning which children should reach appropriate to their age, as they make progress on the short-term objectives.

It is unfortunate, however, that there is no indication of whether practitioners of conductive education would agree to the use of norm-referenced tests for assessing whether children have reached the ultimate goal of orthofunction. Worse still for the present attempt at defining standards to which children should ultimately progress, are other authoritative accounts of what constitutes orthofunction, which are ill-defined, different from, and incompatible with, the above descriptions.

Hari and Tillemans (1984, p.27–28) can be quoted as follows: "Orthofunction is quite difficult to define, but it includes: (i) the integration of what has been learned so far, as separate items; (ii) a person's best performance to date achieved without the use of a by-pass (an aid which replaces, rather than assists, the original function); and (iii) the avoidance of stereotyped, pathological behaviour and the adoption of healthy behaviour . . . orthofunction is what is good and acceptable for a particular person. It is the function that his brain has constructed under the guidance of the conductor in order to cope with his situation. It should be judged on its qualities as a coping mechanism, not in terms of preconceived, socially determined criteria applicable to or derived from the performance of others".

It is difficult to grasp the meaning of points (i) and (iii), and nothing like these vague concepts appear in the earlier, more concrete account (Hari, quoted by Cottam and Sutton, 1968). On the other hand, point (ii) and the latter part of the quote seem incompatible with the earlier quoted expectation of general self-sufficiency in a normal environment. It seems that there are no absolute standards for orthofunction, no requirement for a child to meet normal functional criteria determined by the world at large, indeed there seems to an allowance for different orthofunctional goals for individual children. For example, society in general expects that a six year old child should be able to cope independently with all toileting requirements and six year olds, generally, are able to get to a toilet when they need it, undress, carry out the necessary actions, dress and wash.

However, it would seem that such functional criteria would not have to be met for a child with cerebral palsy to be judged orthofunctional, so long as the child was performing at maximum capability. The above definition seems to rule out the use of any norm-referenced criteria in the definition of orthofunctional goals.

A further series of quotes from Hari and Akos (1988) do not clarify the meaning of orthofunction, are ill-defined in other respects and introduce further incompatible concepts. " . . . an orthofunctional person is characterized by a high level of capacity for varying the ways of achieving goals he is aiming for . . . Not even orthofunctionals are able to satisfy every demand immediately . . . The essential difference between an orthofunctional and a dysfunctional lies not so much in their respective achievements as in how they learn" (p.140–141). In this series of quotes it is suggested that variability in functioning is a hall-mark of orthofunction (another criterion) and then, incompatibly, that current functioning is not a criterion but, rather, an ill-defined 'capacity for learning' is a criterion.

To add to the confusion, the following quotes can be taken from the same publication (Hari and Akos, 1988): " . . . successive failures to succeed in meeting social and biological requirements lie behind dysfunctional personality changes . . . Orthofunction therefore is linked with the successful performance of tasks relating to the biological and social demand . . ." (p.144–145). Another criterion is introduced, this time concerned with personality, and then there is a return to an earlier suggestion that the attainment of orthofunction depends on actual performance not just on a capacity for learning. However, the following definitions are also found: "an orthofunctional person is characterized by a general capacity for adaptation or learning which enables him throughout his life to adjust more and more comprehensively to his natural and social environment and on that general capacity his lifelong development depends" (p.141). "Orthofunction is that protean capacity involving the entire personality enabling an individual to satisfy the biological (and social) demands made upon him. These demands differ greatly, first with age and second according to tradition" (p.140). Here there are references to 'personality' and 'capacity for learning' criteria already discussed, as well as a restatement of the notion that orthofunction involves the attainment of levels of functioning matched to biological and social demands, but the final part of the quote succeeds only in adding to the overall confusion. It is suggested that the demands which a child must meet in order to be declared in the Pető Institute is the absence of wheelchairs and a much quoted criterion for orthofunction is the capability to move from place to place without the use of such a device. A rather different tradition can be found in schools in the United Kingdom, where wheelchairs are provided and their use is not a sign of failure. On the contrary, the ability to cope with a motorised wheelchair is a sign of success for a severely handicapped child. The question arises, could orthofunction encompass the use of wheelchairs for mobility, when it is the tradition for wheelchairs to be provided?

The overall conclusion to be drawn from the above discussion is that the long-term objectives of conductive education cannot be described because the accounts of orthofunction which exist, contain too many ill-defined concepts together with apparently conflicting criteria. The proponents of conductive education should be challenged to define the long-term objectives, including the concept of orthofunction, if only to allow for an independent verification of whether objectives are actually met.

5.4 METHODS USED TO BRING ABOUT DEVELOPMENT

5.4.1 Introduction

Children with cerebral palsy are considered to have a learning disorder, hence, the intervention required is viewed as education rather than treatment or therapy (Hari and Tillemans, 1984). The conductor aims to transform every moment of the day into a learning situation (Szekely, 1975). ". . . Conductive Education does not restrict teaching to particular activities but covers the entire day and all its occupations" (Hari and Akos, 1988; p.155). "Every function demanding a personal contact . . . is an education function, so none thereof must be entrusted to somebody else" (other than a conductor) (Hari, 1975; p.40). Clearly, it is difficult to discuss the methods used in conductive education in detailed and concrete terms when, presumably, every interaction between conductors and children all through the day has a purpose and the nature of each interaction is prescribed by the system.

An advance in describing the method can, however, be made by giving an account of the daily timetable for residential pupils which includes 'the daily schedule', in which is embedded three other categories of activities— 'task series', school programme and 'free time'. In addition, four other features of conductive education can be considered 'methodological'; education in groups only, education by conductors only, the extensive use of so-called 'rhythmical intention', and 'facilitation'. This section will be concluded with an attempt to describe relationships between the methods and objectives of conductive education.

5.4.2   Daily Timetable

5.4.2.1   The Daily Schedule

All postures, postural changes, limb movements and locomotion required for all activities of daily living are performed in ways prescribed by conductive education. Briefly, the sequence begins with getting out of bed then, so called, 'conditioning' ('toilet training') which accustoms the children to using the pot or toilet at set times of the day and in a standard way. There follows a series of breathing and mobility exercises back on the plinth. Then comes dressing and washing of face and hands in a basin followed by walking to breakfast and feeding including learning about food and nutrition. Teeth are brushed before walking back to the 'bedroom' which has now been prepared for the first 'task series' of the day, following which there is the second period of 'conditioning', then washing of hands and a morning snack. The second 'task series' is carried out followed by 'conditioning', washing hands and lunch. The period after lunch may be taken up with another 'task series' or a school programme, followed by 'conditioning', washing hands and tea. There is a further 'task series' before the fifth 'conditioning' for the day after which supper is served. Following teeth cleaning, bathing and final 'conditioning', the children retire to bed. "This routine brings order into the children's lives, accustoming them to a methodical life up to the standard of the requirements for cleanliness and hygiene" (Hari and Akos, 1988; p.153). Furthermore, what has been learned at other times during the day can be put into practice and reinforced in a different context; eg., what has been learned about squatting down and standing up in 'task series' or dressing and undressing in the general daily schedule, can be repeated in the course of 'conditioning'.

5.4.2.2   Task Series

During much of the day and in every activity performed, we require control over our musculo-skeletal system in order to actively maintain steady and stable postures (eg., standing), move from one posture to another (eg., sitting down from a standing posture), reach out, grasp and manipulate objects while maintaining a steady, supportive posture (eg., complicated actions of the upper limbs when seated at a table and feeding), move from place to place (eg., walking) etc. The control we have in carrying out these many individual actions usually emerges spontaneously during development, without the need for specific tuition and the resulting gross-motor and fine-motor skills may, therefore, be termed 'endogenous' (Bairstow, 1983). Children with cerebral palsy, on the other hand, do not have the basic endogenous skills required for postural control, locomotion and hand function. Since the children are viewed as having a learning disorder, the lack of skill is considered to be remediable through appropriate teaching. More generally, the aim of conductive education is to " . . . stimulate a developmental process which would not come about spontaneously" (Hari and Tillemans, 1984; p.20).

As much as six hours in a day is spent on so-called 'task series' aimed specifically at teaching children to gain the basic control over their musculature which normally emerges spontaneously, thereby facilitating the acquisition of other motor skills which depend on the underlying motor repertoire; eg., the skills required for activities of daily living. Each task series is a sequence of actions composed of postures, postural changes, upper limb movements and lower limb movements. " . . . each partial task facilitates the performance of the next and so leads on, step by step, to a goal not immediately within the capability of patients with a specific dysfunction" (Hari and Akos, 1988; p.165). The different task series require control over the musculature of the limbs and trunk in different contexts and with the body in different positions; eg., in one task series the children may be required to stretch their legs and arms while lying down, then in another series they must stretch their limbs while standing up. All postures, postural changes and limb movements making up the task series are to be found in the activities of daily living which form the daily schedule described earlier. "Each day task-series facilitate the satisfaction of all the social and biological requirements comprised in the daily schedule. Day by day the level of achievement required by the schedule rises and indeed is bound to do so when task-series are worked through. This is their justification" (Hari and Akos, 1988; p.165). Hence, the daily schedule, including the education curriculum, is the ultimate goal of the task series.

A particular task series may consist of between twenty and thirty smaller tasks. Although each child in a group carries out the same sequence of tasks, individual differences may be great in as much as each child may complete the tasks in an individual way and there may also be differences in purpose; eg., while turning over, one child may be required to stretch his legs and keep them adducted while another child may be required to support himself on his hands. Children are grouped to minimise disparity in the speed with which partial tasks can be completed. Activities are, however, organised to take into account individual differences in speed so that, as far as possible, faster children are not kept waiting without anything to do while slower children complete a partial task. As goals are achieved, more and more elements are gradually built into task series and the goals are changed; eg., extending the range of conditions in which a partial task can be performed (walking on a rough surface after learning to walk on a smooth surface).

5.4.2.3   School Programme

The school programme includes teaching arithmetic, reading, writing and environmental knowledge and aims to prepare children for studies required in Hungarian primary schools (Hari, 1975). The programme is fully integrated with activities taking place at other times during the day; for example, skills learned in the 'task series' are repeated during the school programme (a child holds up his hand when his name is called, or stands up to answer a question), while something learned in school may be used in 'task series' (counting aloud while performing a partial task).

5.4.2.4   Free Time

There are periods during the day that might provide a break for the group as a whole, or free time for individual children when, for example, a very mobile child manages to complete an activity like walking to the breakfast room and needs to wait while others catch up. The methods of conductive education operate even during such periods. "The children have free time here which must not be taken away from them but, on the contrary, they must be taught, practically without their noticing it, how to use their free time . . . the Conductor is prepared to give them tailor-made help if they need it" (Hari and Akos, 1988; p.151). The day has no gaps or interruptions and the conductor brings the spontaneous activities from free time into the education process. Furthermore, "Break-time is not a break for the Conductor, but almost imperceptibly she channels the spontaneous activity of the children at play" (Hari and Akos, 1988; p.180) so that action patterns developed in 'task series' are employed throughout the day in various contexts.

5.4.3   Group Work

Children work in groups during all parts of the daily timetable. Groups are specifically composed and "must be large enough to permit individual differences and the formation of sub-groups around similarities" (Hari and

Tillemans, 1984; p.25). As far as possible, all children within a group work to one timetable simultaneously, albeit the precise purpose of each activity, the way it is carried out, and the degree of facilitation required vary and the most severely handicapped child carries out activities more slowly and in a modified form. Benefits resulting from the education of children in groups include the following:

Motivation. "The child's motivation is also influenced by the presence in his group of healthy examples with whom to identify" (Hari and Tillemans, 1984; p.19).

Imitation. "Children with similar problems and requiring similar help must by put next to one another. A less active child or one who still has difficulty in understanding what is wanted would be put next to an active child or one who understands it very well, so that he can imitate his neighbour, watching him to see the right thing to do" (Hari and Akos, 1988; p.171).

Attention. Since all activities surrounding a child are of a similar nature to that which the child should be carrying out, there is nothing in the immediate environment which is irrelevant to the current task. Furthermore, "Less attentive children are put among the more attentive" (Hari and Akos, 1988; p.171) in order to facilitate an individual's attention. Each child is made to feel responsible to the group and is therefore not inclined to be disruptive.

Reinforcement. The success of individual children is noted by conductors and is rewarded with praise from the group as a whole. "Keeping to the schedule, successfully completing a task, and the success of every individual member become matters of general concern . . ." (Hari and Akos, 1988; p.208).

Interpersonal Development. "A group is the principle vehicle for interpersonal relations . . . the group is seen as an essential part of the practice of Conductive Education" (Hari and Akos, 1988; p.205).

5.4.4 Conductor

Two key methodological issues determine the role played by conductors and the way in which they carry out their work. First, conductive education is a " . . . unified system and that its concepts form a unitary whole . . . its details can never be separated . . . is directed at the whole, not to improve symptoms merely but the whole personality" (Hari and Akos, 1988; p.214). Having one type of professional—the conductor—whose role is to put "into effect the entire system of requirements for living" (Hari and Akos, 1988; p.215) is the main method for ensuring that the capabilities and difficulties of individual children are considered holistically during their education. "Fragmentation of the child . . . is avoided by making the conductor the contact person . . . " (Hari and Tillemans, 1984; p.20). Second, conductive education requires good interpersonal relationships between conductors and children and this is achieved by having conductors work in groups with the children. Tasks are shared among the conductors, and the children see the conductors working as a team rather than as individuals. This " . . . diminishes tension . . . between a Conductor and individual dysfunctionals . . .each child has less of a feeling of being the centre of the Conductor's attention and yet it is obvious to every child that the Conductor is paying attention to him and is helping him if necessary" (Hari and Akos, 1988; p.208).

5.4.5   Rhythmical Intention

"In practice, rhythmical intention goes like this. The Conductor defines a goal, for example, 'I raise my right arm' or 'I lie down on my back'. The members of the group repeat the statement of the goal and then carry it out, counting out aloud, 'One, two, three, four, five'. The entire group counts together" (Hari and Akos, 1988; p.209). Rhythmic intention is used extensively throughout the day and especially in 'task series' (Section 5.4.2.2), and serves the following functions:

Goal Setting   A goal is made conscious and explicit by having it verbally stated. Furthermore, "Verbal intention prepares the action and starts it off in all its complexity" (Hari and Akos, 1988; p.209). "The words must express what the child is to think" (Hari and Tillemans, 1984; p.31).

Regulation.   "If we begin counting out aloud and stop suddenly, people around us will go on counting involuntarily in their own minds. The sequence of numbers virtually forces itself on us and that is precisely why counting forms a convenient vehicle for rhythm. . . . By rhythmical intention a Conductor makes a group set up a rhythm and this rhythm which we know to have such an energizing significance takes effect amplified into a chorus. . . . counting has a co-ordinating role in filing out the rather lengthy period between verbally intending a task and accomplishing it" (Hari and Akos, 1988; p.209–210). Singing and reciting nursery rhymes are other ways of maintaining rhythm.

Active Involvement.   Rhythmical intention is always carried out in the 'first person'. "This helps to underline the fact that the child (repeating the 'I') is the principle actor in the scene" (Hari and Tillemans, 1984; p.31)—it serves to involve the child in his own education.

Attention.   The scope for attending to anything else but the immediate task is severely limited when verbalization and performance are closely linked.

Group Work. "Rhythmical intention in a chorus also means that the members of a group have to work together and co-operate regularly, however great the differences between them . . . rhythmical intention facilitates not only the learning of an activity but also the cohesion of the group" (Hari and Akos, 1988; p.210).

Interpersonal Development. "From the point of co-operation within a group, rhythmical intention is important . . . because it facilitates caring for one another" (Hari and Akos, 1988; p.211); ie., when children verbalize a goal or count out aloud, it is believed that they do so not only for their own benefit but for the benefit of others in the group.

Speech. ". . . Motor and speech development have to be planned as a unit" (Hari and Tillemans, 1984; p.28). Rhythmical intention ". . . forms an introduction to learning to speak and the first signs of it may appear precisely through rhythmical intention" (Hari and Akos, 1988; p.211).

5.4.6 Facilitation

Conductive education requires all children, regardless of individual differences, to participate actively in, and complete, all parts of the daily schedule, task series and school programme set for the group. Conductive education also requires incremental improvement in the children day-by-day; "yesterday's result . . . is not good enough for today" (Hari and Akos, 1988; p.171). The method used to achieve these dual requirements is 'facilitation' and the gradual withdrawal thereof.

"The process of facilitation for us has an educational . . . connotation. Facilitation meets every condition necessary for a dysfunctional to be able to carry out an activity through his own efforts" (Hari and Akos, 1988; p.186). It serves partly to provide a "way of completing whatever they have to do and partly to ensure that every member of the group keeps pace in working together" (Hari and Akos, 1988; p.195). It also performs a corrective function so that a child's activities are progressively shaped. "Facilitation can be used before starting a task . . . during and after it . . ." (Hari and Akos, 1988; p.200) and a major role of the conductor is to employ various means of facilitation to commence, continue and complete every activity.

The setting of explicit and immediate goals by the conductor and the use of verbal intention are ways of facilitating the initiation of a task.

There are numerous ways of facilitating performance once a task is underway: rhythmical intention; carefully structuring task series so that each partial task facilitates the performance of the next; positioning the child so that gravity will assist the child to extend a limb, for example; employing ladder-backed chairs and slatted plinths to enable a child to be stabilized while learning to gain control; having the children work in groups—"Their companions' success is another important form of facilitation. It stimulates both imitation and greater originality" (Hari and Akos, 1988; p.194); the creation by the conductor of a favourable atmosphere for the task—"This general effect depended exclusively on the interpersonal relationship" (Hari and Akos, 1988; p.204). The most noticeable method of facilitating performance, however, is the individual physical help a conductor may give to a child. "Conductors aim at maximum independence: they seek to avoid holding the child or supporting him. They *will* assist when failure would otherwise be inevitable. Credit for accomplishment, however, should go to the child, not the conductor" (Hari and Tillemans, 1984; p.20). ". . . when a child has begun a movement but cannot go beyond the half-way point and . . . failure is imminent, the conductor must help the child to succeed by offering a minimum of appropriate help, thus preventing a sense of failure and allowing him to give himself credit for the completion of the learning task" (Hari and Tillemans, 1984; p.27). But, the conductors ". . . help the child in areas that are not central to the learning task . . . Any support used in carrying out a movement should be just an aid. . . . to stretch joints, to stabilise body-parts not essential to the process of learning, and to free or control movement in body-parts which are central to learning" (Hari and Tillemans, 1984; p.29–30).

The principal method of facilitation employed after a task is completed is the careful noting by the conductor of a child's progress and success and verbalizing this to the child and to the group as a whole.

As time goes by the ". . . extent or proportion of the task achieved will increase naturally . . ." (Hari and Akos, 1988; p.193). The "degree of facilitation needed grows less from day to day" (Hari and Akos, 1988; p.174) and "gradually becomes superfluous" (Hari and Akos, 1988; p.186). Moreover, the conductor must gradually withdraw facilitation, for example, withdrawing rhythmical intention (Hari and Akos, 1988; p.210), and this is the main method for ensuring that children become more independent. "The task, though chosen by the conductor . . . in the course of time becomes the child's personal responsibility. In the learning-teaching session the conductor has to fade more and more into the background, the child increasingly occupying the centre of the stage" (Hari and Tillemans, 1984; p.31).

5.4.7   Relationships Between Methods and Objectives

The immediate aims of conductive education cover the following domains: social behaviour, upper-limb function, self-care, position changing, walking, speech and communication, and cognition. It is difficult to say whether parts of the daily timetable, group work, the conductor, rhythmical intention and facilitation are more relevant to some aims than others. "If we were to attempt to isolate the principal features of Conductive Education we would have to point out as the first one that its details can never be separated, for if we neglect one thing the whole suffers" (Hari and Akos, 1988; p.214).

Aspects of upper limb functioning, position changing and walking are focused on intensively during 'task series' but are also the subject of teaching during the daily schedule, school programme and supervised activities during 'free-time'. Furthermore, group work, rhythmical intention and facilitation are all used to promote motor functioning.

Interpersonal skills required for progress along the social scales are constantly being fostered throughout the daily timetable because children are required to interact with one-another in group-work, with the conductors generally and when rhythmical intention is being employed.

Skills required for speech and communication are fostered during the daily schedule by the use of rhythmical intention during task series and are also fostered during the school programme.

Abilities required for progress along the attention, motivation and learning abilities scales are constantly being promoted by group work, rhythmical intention and the gradual withdrawal of facilitation.

Finally, close supervision of the daily schedule according to the methods of conductive education is the means by which skills relevant to self-care are promoted, although 'task-series' are also relevant because they are concerned with the development of endogenous types of skills which are basic requirements for the daily schedule.

In general, there is a strong emphasis on viewing the children holistically, keeping all teaching objectives constantly on the agenda and using each teaching opportunity to promote many aspects of function simultaneously.

Nothing can be said about methods used to bring about long-term orthofunctional goals, until such goals have been defined (Section 5.3).

5.5   PRINCIPLES OF CONDUCTIVE EDUCATION

There seem to be rules in conductive education which have general relevance and operate throughout the day regardless of specific objectives. The rules can be thought of as the principles of conductive education *in practice* and the following discussion is an attempt to distil the rules from Section 5.4 and from the following publications; Akos (1975), Hari and Akos (1988) and Hari and Tillemans (1984). They can be categorised according to whether they apply primarily to the children, the conductors or the implementation of conductive education. The generation of hypotheses concerning which principles are crucial to the effective implementation of conductive education must await a demonstration that conductive education is effective.

5.5.1 Rules Applying to the Children

The following general attitudes are expected in the children and are continually fostered by conductive education:

i. Personal responsibility and commitment to learning such that the child must wish to participate and solve problems.

ii. Expectation of hard-work, perserverance and incremental improvement, with the child knowing that 'yesterday's result is not good enough for today'.

iii. Positive attitudes and expectations regarding their own progress and long term future.

iv. Responsibility for the welfare of other children in the group.

5.5.2 Rules Applying to the Conductors

The following general attitudes and practices are expected in the conductors:

i. Positive attitudes and expectations regarding progress in the children.

ii. Creation of favourable learning opportunities, the means for success and the means for preventing failure.

iii. Demonstrating to the children that nothing but hard work and greater independence is acceptable.

iv. Fostering in the children the belief that success comes only from personal effort.

v. Use of reinforcement—prompt positive comments to individual children for success and progress, never negative comments for unwanted or inappropriate behaviour but only suggestions for different activity.

vi. Responsibility to other conductors in the group in fostering team work.

5.5.3 Rules in the Implementation of Conductive Education

The following seem to be general rules which apply when conductive education is implemented:

i. Since movement is considered to be a contributor to learning, children must be as active as possible throughout the day.

ii.   Conductive education covers the whole day which is marked by routine and order, with a constant flow of activities and no gaps, but optimally paced so that no child is overloaded and every child is given time to complete all activities.

iii.   All activities are carried out in parallel while working in groups, but individual goals, methods of facilitation and levels of attainment are devised.

iv.   All activities are goal orientated. The goals are defined in terms of what the child requires for the longer-term future and the goals are always made explicit to the child.

v.   Activities throughout the day and from day-to-day are inter-related. They form a longitudinal series and their relevance to one another is made explicit to the children. Activities are used in which underlying abilities are embedded, rather than activities which focus on abilities separately.

vi.   All children must be actively engaged in succeeding in all activities and this requires the optimal use of facilitation by the conductors. Circumstances for success must be provided so that all verbally intended goals are achieved.

vii.   Most objectives are concerned with the progressive acquisition of independence from physical and personal assistance and this is achieved by the gradual withdrawal of facilitation.

viii. Loss of attention, loss of motivation or fatigue are indicators of absence of learning and, therefore, the need to introduce novelty or to increase difficulty so that interest and attention are regained. Straight repetition, fatigue or loss of attention must be avoided.

ix.   Cerebral palsy is considered to be a learning disorder, hence the disorder must be overcome as far as possible with conductive education before any physical disability is treated. ". . . rehabilitation of the motor disorder should be followed by that of the motor disability. This sequence must not be reversed" (Hari, 1975; p.44). For example, there seems to be a reluctance to allow early surgical intervention as a prophylaxis, but such intervention is permitted later as a corrective measure.

5.6   CONCLUSIONS

Although conductive education has existed in Hungary for around 40 years and has been the focus of attention of an increasing number of professionals in the United Kingdom for around 30 years, no clear and comprehensive accounts of the objectives, methods and principles of conductive education have been published in English by proponents of the system. The present account has relied on English translations of Hungarian text, endorsed by the original authors who were associated with the Pető Institute. While allowing for lack of fidelity in translation, it is difficult not to be critical of the available publications.

Key features of the system are not well explained; eg., all goals in task series are verbalised by all members of a group in unison yet individual differences in purpose are somehow allowed for; given that children vary in their speed of learning and performance, it is difficult to envisage how group work in which children must carry out activities strictly in parallel can be maintained without holding up 'quick' children or allowing 'slow' children to fall behind; it is important that children remain interested and motivated throughout the day but it is unclear how this is achieved when all activities are group activities and no allowance seems to be made for individual interests.

Many statements and beliefs seem never to have been challenged or tested; eg., conductive education stimulates a developmental process; negative comments for unwanted or inappropriate behaviour should never be made; verbal intention causes a child to think explicitly about a goal; rhythmical intention limits the scope for a child attending to anything else but the immediate task.

Many assertions seem unbelievable; eg., dysfunction is a personality problem and conductive education is directed at improving the whole personality (Section 5.3) yet it is difficult to believe that the manifestations of cerebral palsy are due to a personality problem and conductive education would seem to constrain the development of individual personality since children do not have the benefit of unstructured or unsupervised time in which they can express their individuality; straight repetition of activities must be avoided (Section 5.5.3) yet repetition in the highly structured daily timetable is a noticeable feature of conductive education; task series are directly relevant to activities in the daily schedule and all children understand their relevance (Section 5.5.3) yet any young child, especially one with low general cognitive ability, could not be expected to understand the relationship between widely separated activities; activities are optimally paced so that no child is overloaded (Section 5.5.3) yet a common complaint voiced by parents is the fatique experienced by their children.

There are examples of text which contain apparently conflicting statements; eg., other children's success stimulates both imitation and greater originality (Section 5.4.6).

There are examples of incorrect use of terminology some of which are fundamental; eg., cerebral palsy is considered to be a *learning disorder* (Section 5.4.1., Section 5.5.3) yet some children have a low general cognitive ability (ie., a learning disorder) but also have physical disabilities which need early surgical correction, while other children have a high general cognitive ability (ie., no learning disorder) but have no expressive language due to a disorder of the speech apparatus.

Finally, there are poorly defined terms which are used frequently; eg., orthofunction.

The extent to which the present account of conductive education is clear and coherent is more a function of careful choice and juxtaposition of quotations than of clarity and coherence of the original texts which are singularly frustrating in their opacity and confusion. The above examples chosen for criticism have been taken from the present review and it is not difficult to find even more problematic examples elsewhere in the publications. On the other hand, selecting and juxtaposing quotations in order to distil meaning is bound to introduce distortions and it is unlikely that the Pető Institute would endorse the principles of conductive education listed here. Proponents of conductive education should meet the challenge of providing a clear and comprehensive account of the system in English, which is the language understood by the majority of the world's scientific community, as a first step in having the system widely accepted.

Given the difficulties in identifying the principles of conductive education, it proved impossible to identify which of the implied principles might be crucial to its effective implementation.

Appendix 5.1

SCALES DESIGNED BY CONDUCTORS FROM THE PETŐ INSTITUTE FOR MEASURING THE PROGRESS CHILDREN MAKE AS THEY ATTAIN CONDUCTIVE EDUCATION GOALS

Social behaviour: Formal group role (eg. class situation)

8. Takes leading role in a large group (eg., group of 8 children)

7. Takes leading role in a small group (eg., group of 3 children)

6. Does not take a leading role in a group, but participates in group activity and shows the potential to lead.

5. Does not take a leading role in a group, but participates in group activity and does *not* show the potential to lead.

4. Does not work within a group, but shows the potential for group work.

3. Does not work within a group, does not show the potential for group work, but the group wants to accept the child.

2. Does not work within a group, does not show the potential for group work, and the group is not willing to accept the child.

1. _____

Social behaviour: Relationship with adults

8. Does establish good relationship with parents and other adults generally.

7. Does establish good relationship with only a few adults (eg., only those who care for the child), but shows the potential for broader contact.

6. Does establish good relationship with only a few adults (eg., only those who care for the child), and does *not* show the potential for broader contact.

5. Does establish good relationship with only a few adults (eg., only those who care for the child), but not easily or readily.

4. Does establish good relationship with parents only, does not accept other adults or strangers, but does show the potential for contact.

3.   Does establish good relationship with parents only, does not accept other adults or strangers, and does not show the potential for contact.

2.   Does establish good relationship with one adult only (eg., one parent, or a caregiver).

1.   Does not establish good relationship of any kind with any adult, even within the family.

Social behaviour: Relationship with children in play or family situation

8.   Does establish good reciprocal relationship with other children, including children outside the family, regardless of their age.

7.   Does establish good reciprocal relationship with other children, including children outside the family, but only with children of a particular age.

6.   Does establish good reciprocal relationship with children within the family, but not generally with children outside the family, although does show the potential for such general contact.

5.   Does establish good reciprocal relationship with children within the family, but with only one child outside the family.

4.   Does establish good reciprocal relationship with children within the family, but not with even one child outside the family although does show the potential for such contact.

3.   Does establish good reciprocal relationship with children, but only within the family.

2.   Does not establish good reciprocal relationship with children within the family, but does show the potential for such contact.

1.   Does not establish good reciprocal relationship with children within the family, and does *not* show any potential for such contact.

Social behaviour: Initiating individual contact with other people

8.   Readily initiates contact with adults or other children, and readily accepts such contact.

7.   Occasionally initiates contact with adults or other children, and readily accepts such contact.

6.   Rarely initiates contact with adults or other children, but readily accepts such contact.

5.   Only readily accepts contact with adults or other children.

4.   Occasionally accepts contact with adults or other children.

3.   Rarely accepts contact with adults or other children, and generally rejects contact.

2.   Generally rejects contact with adults or other children.

1.   Generally indifferent to any attempt to establish contact, but occasionally shows interest or a response, and therefore shows potential for contact.

Upper limb function (left limb): Differentiated movements of fingers

8.   Does manipulate and does use a variety of objects with the hand, employing all fingers appropriately.

7.   Does manipulate and does use a variety of objects with the hand, employing all fingers appropriately, but slowly or clumsily.

6.   Does manipulate and does use a variety of objects with the hand, but only using the thumb and some fingers well.

5.   Does manipulate and does use objects with the hand, but only some objects or with limited power.

4.   Does show some differentiated movements of one or more fingers, but does *not* oppose the thumb with any finger and does not grip any object with a pincer grip.

3.   No differentiated movements of any finger.

2.   _____

1.   _____

Upper limb function (right limb): Reaching

8.   Does reach freely in a variety of directions, regardless of support or seating position.

7. Does reach freely in a variety of directions, but only in a particular position or supported in a particular way. *OR*, only reaches freely in few directions without support.

6. Only reaches freely in few directions with support. *OR*, reaches freely in only one direction without support.

5. Only reaches forward with support and sliding the arm on the surface of the table, and does maintain the final extended position.

4. Only reaches forward, and does not maintain the final extended position.

3. Starts to initiate a reaching movement, with support and with manual assistance.

2. Does not initiate any form of reaching movement, even with maximal support and assistance.

1. _____

Upper limb function (left limb): Reaching

8. Does reach freely in a variety of directions, regardless of support or seating position.

7. Does reach freely in a variety of directions, but only if in a particular position or supported in a particular way. *OR*, only reaches freely in few directions without support.

6. Only reaches freely in few directions with support. *OR*, reaches freely in only one direction without support.

5. Only reaches forward with support and sliding the arm on the surface of the table, and does maintain the final extended position.

4. Only reaches forward, and does not maintain the final extended position.

3. Starts to initiate a reaching movement, with support and with manual assistance.

2. Does not initiate any form of reaching movement, even with maximal support and assistance.

1. _____

Upper limb function (right limb): Holding an object

8.   Does independently grasp, hold and release a variety of objects readily and in any circumstance.

7.   Does independently grasp, hold and release a variety of objects readily but with difficulty, or only in particular circumstances (eg., with support).

6.   Does independently grasp, hold and release only particular objects readily.

5.   Does independently grasp and hold objects, but releases them only with difficulty.

4.   Does independently grasp and hold objects, but does not release them.

3.   Does independently grasp a particular object, but does not maintain the grasp.

2.   Does grasp a particular object but only if it is placed in the hand.

1.   Does not grasp or hold any object even if placed within the hand.

Upper limb function (left limb): Holding an object

8.   Does independently grasp, hold and release a variety of objects readily and in any circumstance.

7.   Does independently grasp, hold and release a variety of objects readily but with difficulty, or only in particular circumstances (eg., with support).

6.   Does independently grasp, hold and release only particular objects readily.

5.   Does independently grasp and hold objects, but releases them only with difficulty.

4.   Does independently grasp and hold objects, but does not release them.

3.   Does independently grasp a particular object, but does not maintain the grasp.

2.   Does grasp a particular object but only if it is placed in the hand.

1.   Does not grasp or hold any object even if placed within the hand.

Self-care: Dressing (putting on and taking off clothes and footwear)

8.   Does independently put on and take off all items of clothing and footwear (shoes and socks).

7.   Does independently put on and take off all items of clothing and footwear, but untidily or with errors.

6.   Does independently put on and take off all items of clothing but needs help with footwear.

5.   Does independently put on and take off only some items of clothing in unprotected situation. *OR*, does independently put on and take off most items of clothing but only in protected situation.

4.   Does independently take off clothing only, and needs assistance to put on clothing.

3.   Does independently take off only a few items of clothing, and generally needs assistance for dressing and undressing.

2.   Needs assistance for all of undressing and dressing, and participates in the activities.

1.   Needs assistance for all of undressing and dressing, and does not participate in the activities.

Self-care: Shoe-laces

8.   Does independently and correctly tie shoe laces of various kinds, in a variety of positions, and does untie laces independently.

7.   Does independently tie shoe laces of various kinds, in a variety of positions, but slowly or clumsily, and does untie laces independently.

6.   Does independently tie shoelaces of various kinds, but only in a particular position, and does untie laces independently.

5.   Does independently tie shoelaces only of a particular kind, and does untie laces independently.

4.   Does not independently tie any sort of shoelace, but does untie independently.

3.   Does not independently tie or untie shoelaces.

2.   _____

1.   _____

Self-care: Buttons

8.   Does independently do up and undo buttons of various kinds in a variety of positions.

7.   Does independently do up and undo buttons of various kinds but slowly or clumsily, and in a variety of positions.

6.   Does independently do up and undo buttons of various kinds but only in a particular position.

5.   Does independently do up and undo buttons but only of a particular kind.

4.   Does not independently do up buttons, but does independently undo them.

3.   Does not independently do up or undo buttons.

2.   _____

1.   _____

Self-care: Feeding

8.   Does independently eat a variety of food using a variety of cutlery without making a mess.

7.   Does independently eat a variety of food using a variety of cutlery, but clumsily or making a mess.

6.   Does independently eat a variety of food, but only with a normal spoon without making a mess.

5.   Does independently eat a variety of food, but only with a special spoon without making a mess, *or* a normal spoon and making a mess.

4.   Does independently eat with fingers only, and requires assistance for eating with a spoon.

3. Needs assistance to eat with fingers, and does not use any form of cutlery for eating.

2. Does not participate in feeding itself, but does take in, chew and swallow a variety of food.

1. Does not participate in feeding itself, and only takes in special food.

Self-care: Toileting

8. Does use toilet independently and uses paper independently and no need for adult supervision.

7. Does use toilet independently, does not need potty, but needs adult supervision for use of toilet paper.

6. Does use potty or toilet independently. Indicates need reliably. Nappies not used.

5. Requires special aid, but does use it independently. Indicates need reliably. Nappies not used.

4. Requires special aid, and requires assistance to use it. Indicates need reliably. Nappies not used.

3. Requires special aid, and requires assistance. Does indicate need but not reliably. Nappies required sometimes (eg., at night).

2. Requires special aid, and requires assistance. Does not indicate the need, but does indicate the action. Nappies always required.

1. Requires special aid, and requires assistance. Does not indicate either the need or the action. Nappies always required.

Position changing: Standing up from a stool, and sitting down to a stool

7. Does independently stand-up and sit-down, and does not hold on to anything.

6. Does independently stand-up and sit-down, but holds on to something.

5. Does independently stand-up and sit-down, holding or supporting on something fixed, and requires verbal instruction.

4.   Requires assistance with either standing up or sitting down while holding on to something, and requires assistance with the legs *or* the arms.

3.   Requires assistance with both standing up and sitting down while holding on to something, and requires assistance with both legs *and* arms.

2.   Does not stand-up or sit-down even with assistance, but attempts to try.

1.   Does not stand-up or sit-down even with assistance and does not attempt to try.

Position changing: Standing up from the floor, and sitting down to the floor

8.   Does independently stand-up and sit-down, and does not hold on to anything.

7.   Does independently stand-up and sit-down, but holds on to something.

6.   Does independently stand-up and sit-down, holding on to something, and requires verbal instruction.

5.   Does independently stand-up holding on to something and with verbal instruction, but requires assistance for sitting down.

4.   Requires assitance with both standing up and sitting down while holding on to something, but assistance only with the legs *or* the arms.

3.   Requires assistance with both standing up and sitting down while holding on to something, and requires assistance with both legs *and* arms.

2.   Does not stand-up or sit-down even with assistance, but attempts to try.

1.   Does not stand-up or sit-down even with assistance and does not attempt to try.

Position changing: Sitting up from supine, sitting, lying down to supine on the plinth

	Sit-up		Lie-down		Sit
8	Independent.* Not holding on.** No verbal instr.	(and)	Independent. Not holding on. No verbal instr.	(and)	Independent. Not holding on. No verbal instr.
7	Independent. Grasping or pulling. No verbal instr.	(or)	Independent. Grasping or pulling. No verbal instr.	(and)	Independent. Not holding on. No verbal instr.
6	Independent. Grasping or pulling Verbal instr.	(or)	Independent. Grasping or pulling. Verbal instr.	(and)	Independent. Not holding on. No verbal instr.
5	Requires part assistance.	(or)	Requires part assistance.	(and)	Independent. Not holding on. No verbal instr.
4	Requires part assistance.	(or)	Requires part assistance.	(and)	Requires assistance or holding on.
3	Lifts head independently but requires assistance for all the rest.	(and)	Requires assistance for all.	(and)	Requires assistance or holding on.
2	Requires assistance for all but attempting to participate.	(and)	Requires assistance for all but attempting to participate.	(and)	Requires assistance but attempting to participate.
1	Requires assistance and not attempting.	(and)	Requires assistance and not attempting.	(and)	Requires assistance and not attempting.

* means independent of assistance from another person.
** means no need to hold on to any physical aid.

Positing changing: Rolling 360 degrees on the floor commencing from supine

7.   Does independently roll 360° in both directions with ease and maintains the correct path.

6.   Does independently roll 360° but slowly or clumsily, or does not maintain the correct path in both directions.

5.   Does independently roll 180° but does not continue because the limbs are placed incorrectly.

4.   Does independently roll 90° and requires assistance to complete the actions.

3.   Does independently start the action (eg., turns the head, or reaches across with the arm), but requires assistance for most of the action.

2.   Does *not* independently perform any part of the action, but attempts to participate.

1.   Does *not* independently perform any part of the action, and does *not* attempt to participate.

Walking: Without aids and bare-foot

11.   Does walk independently on a variety of surfaces, with normal speed.

10.   Does walk independently on a variety of surfaces, but is walking insecurely; eg., problems with changing direction, changing speed, stepping around an obstacle.

9.   Does walk independently on plane surface only, with normal speed.

8.   Does walk independently on plane surface only, but only in protected situation and slow speed, or only to a defined goal.

7.   Does walk independently but only for a few steps, or does stand independently.

6.   Does *not* walk independently for even one step, or does not stand independently.

Walking: With aids (eg., personal assistance, furniture, sticks)

10. Does walk independently with one stick on a variety of surfaces, with normal speed.

9. Does walk independently with two sticks on a variety of surfaces, with normal speed.

8. Does walk independently with two sticks on plane surface, and slowly.

7. Does walk independently with two sticks, but only indoors and for limited distance.

6. Does walk independently but only between parallel bars, or between two chairs, or behind a chair pushing it.

5. Does walk independently but only between parallel bars, or between two chairs, or behind a chair, **and** with verbal instruction.

4. Does walk but only between parallel bars, or between two chairs, or behind a chair, **and** requires help from one person to move the arms or the legs.

3. Does walk but only between parallel bars, or between two chairs, or behind a chair, **and** requires help from **two** persons.

2. Does **not** participate in walking but attempts to try.

1. Does **not** participate in walking and not attempting to try.

Speech and communication: Speech

8. Correct sentence construction and clear pronunciation of words.

7. Correct sentence construction, unclear pronunciation, but understandable.

6. Construction of short sentences, and severe problems with pronunciation.

5. Uses only individual words, no sentences, severe problems with pronunciation.

4. Pronounces only parts of words when attempting to speak.

3.   Makes sounds (not parts of words) when attempting to speak.

2.   Does not attempt to speak, but does make a variety of sounds otherwise.

1.   Does not attempt to speak, and makes no sounds other than crying.

Speech and communication: Communication (verbal and non-verbal)

8.   Does verbally communicate above age level.

7.   Does verbally communicate appropriately for age.

6.   If communicating only non-verbally, does communicate appropriately for age.

5.   Does verbally or non-verbally communicate but below age level.

4.   Does verbally or non-verbally communicate more than a few immediate needs but poorly.

3.   Does verbally communicate only a few immediate needs.

2.   Does non-verbally communicate only a few immediate needs.

1.   Does not communicate anything.

Cognition: General knowledge

8.   Above average knowledge of personal and impersonal circumstances.

7.   Average knowledge of personal and impersonal circumstances.

6.   Below average knowledge of personal and impersonal circumstances.

5.   Average knowledge of personal circumstances only.

4.   Below average knowledge of personal circumstances only.

3.   Poor knowledge of immediate personal circumstances.

2.   Knowledge only of immediate personal requirements.

1.   _____

Cognition: Attention

8.   Above average quality of attention in group work.

7.   Average quality of attention in group work.

6.   Easy to distract, or spontaneously changes attention in group work.

5.   Directs attention only for short time in group work. *OR*, inappropriately fixes attention.

4.   Can attend in a small group only, and only for particular tasks or in a restricted environment.

3.   Can attend only if there is one-to-one contact with another person in a restricted environment.

2.   Attention can be attracted only for brief moments.

1.   Attention can be attracted only by a close caregiver for a few specific purposes.

Cognition: Learning ability

8.   Does learn something new quickly, and uses it with previously learned material.

7.   Does learn something new with average speed, and uses it with previously learned material.

6.   Does learn something new but slowly, and requires special help for learning.

5.   Does learn something new, but does not use it with previously learned material, and does not understand the connection between different knowledge.

4.   Does learn something new, but only something very particular and with repetition (eg., rhymes or songs).

3.   Does learn something very simple, but only with much repetition, and requires repetition to retain it (otherwise forgotten).

2.   _____

1.   _____

Cognition: Motivation

8.   Self-motivated strongly and above age level in many different tasks.

7.   Self-motivated, age appropriate, in many different tasks.

6.   Good, self-motivation in particular areas, but poor in other areas.

5.   Poor self-motivation, and generally requires external encouragement to perform any task.

4.   Poor self-motivation, and can be motivated only in tasks connected with immediate personal comfort and needs.

3.   Very difficult to motivate to do any other task not already spontaneously performing.

2.   _____

1.   _____

Effectiveness of Conductive Education Compared to the Effectiveness of United Kingdom Special Education (Objective 3)

6.1 INTRODUCTION

Objective 3 required a study of the effectiveness of conductive education for children with cerebral palsy in the Birmingham Institute, compared to the effectiveness of some alternative British programmes. A battery of assessments suitable for measuring functional and physical characteristics of children with cerebral palsy had to be assembled. The method by which the Birmingham group was selected needed to be documented and their functional abilities established using the battery of assessments. A methodology for identifying a comparison group had to be devised and matching of the groups confirmed with a subset of the assessment battery. It was necessary to compare the groups on a range of collateral data including, family background, formal timetable of the education programmes, attendance of the children, relevance of the assessment battery to the programmes of education and input outside the programmes having possible effects on development. A comparison between the two groups of children in their development had to be carried out and results interpreted in the light of the collateral data. This section reports the methodologies and findings relevant to this objective.

6.2 ASSESSMENT BATTERY

6.2.1 Introduction

Given the predictions outlined in Section 3.7 it was necessary to assess a wide range of functional abilities, and dealing with children with cerebral palsy, it was also necessary to record a range of physical variables. Assessments were needed to cover the following domains: cognitive functioning and academic skills; communication and speech; fine-motor and gross-motor functioning; social behaviour; daily living skills; physical status. The battery assembled, was specifically tailored neither to conductive education nor to United Kingdom special education but collateral data were collected to confirm whether bias in the relevance of the battery to the specific programmes had been avoided. The assessments were concerned with general changes in the children resulting from possible programme-specific gains and, therefore, had to be responsive to changes in the children (Rosenbaum et al, 1985).

There is a problem in assessing children with cerebral palsy in that most published tests for children, have been devised for the non-disabled population. Assessments, in general, need to be designed so that performance reflects ability in a particular domain and is unaffected by abilities in other domains. This is difficult to achieve when, for example, a motor disability can interfere with the expression of cognitive abilities and social skills. Every effort had to be made to disentangle the various domains in the testing situation; eg. using tests of motor functioning which were not cognitively demanding, using tests of cognitive functioning which were, as far as possible, unaffected by motor or language problems.

Some published tests, which had been designed and normed with non-disabled children, could be applied to children in the present study. This was useful since the test items were constructed for children operating in a non-adapted environment. It was possible, therefore, to collect norm-referenced data allowing for an examination of Prediction 3 (Section 3.7), ie. conductive education would enable children to function within a minimally adapted social and physical environment. The tests could also be employed as criterion-referenced instruments by utilising raw scores only.

It was not, however, possible to rely entirely on published tests. It was sometimes necessary to modify existing tests and also to devise completely new tests. The criterion-referenced data thus obtained were sufficient for an examination of Predictions 1 and 2 (Section 3.7). Tests were modified or devised with the aim of creating interval scales of measurement and to have consistency among scales so that an increase in raw score always indicated improvement.

There may be room for argument about whether all the test scores employed, constitute interval level data, or an acceptable approximation to it. On the other hand, similar doubts apply to test scores in almost any context, and yet the interval level assumption is very commonly made. For example, the maximum mark on each question in a school examination is often only assumed to be an interval measure of relative difficulty, and this assumption is necessary if the obtained marks on the questions are to be summed for an overall examination result. Furthermore, two candidates with equal results are usually considered to be equal in achievement because of interval level assumptions, yet they will differ at least quali-tatively if their marks on individual questions were different, and they may even differ quantitatively if the relative difficulty of the questions has not been established on an interval scale.

On the assumption that present test scores constitute interval level data, statistical analyses for the purpose of examining Predictions 1, 2 and 3 (Section 3.7), were based on parametric tests of significance. The alterna-tive assumption (ie., that the test scores are only ordinal) would have required the use of significance tests of lower power than parametric tests (ie., nonparametric tests). If the test scores were assumed from the outset to be ordinal, when in fact they approximate to interval, there would be a risk that significant results be overlooked. The following rule was followed in all statistical analyses: if, on using parametric tests on the basis of the interval level assumption, significant results were obtained close to the threshold of being not significant, less powerful nonparametric tests appropriate to ordinal level data were employed to see if significant results still emerged.

Different methods were used to gather data on the children; ie. direct testing in a one-to-one situation, indirect testing using semi-structured interviews with parents, semi-structured interviews with staff involved with the education of the children and questionnaires sent out to parents. Some domains (eg. social behaviour, daily living skills) were best assessed indirectly (Blake et al, 1985; Law and Letts, 1989) using interviewing techniques, while others (eg. motor) could be assessed both directly and indirectly. Any method of assessment has advantages and disadvantages and employing a range of methods for one domain (where possible) enabled the child to be assessed from different perspectives thus providing a check on whether there was agreement between different sources of information; eg. whether similar results for the motor domain were obtained by interviewing parents, interviewing staff and by direct testing.

Assessments were carried out under partially 'blind' conditions which helped to ensure they were unprejudiced. It was not possible to conceal the identity of the children from those carrying out the assessments but information about any other test result was effectively unavailable. At the time of testing or at the time of interview it was usual to record the performance only, and the child's score was calculated or derived at a later time. Generally, scores could not be affected by other results; eg. staff generally did not know what happened at a previous assessment of a child because previous records were not consulted and could not be remembered; staff did not know the results of other current assessments of a child because different staff were involved with different parts of the assessment and the other results were not available.

Most direct assessments were video-recorded and data were derived from the recordings using written methodologies and criteria. The video-recordings provide a permanent record of children's performance and allowed for checks on inter-observer and intra-observer consistency.

The following sections give a detailed account of the assessment battery and the methodologies employed. Each section relates to a specific assessment and there is an account of what the assessment covers; some assessments cover more than one data domain while others assess only one aspect of a domain. There is also an account of how the assessment was carried out, how raw criterion-referenced scores were calculated, how norm-referenced scores were obtained, and how criterion-referenced data were combined to reduce the size of the data set.

6.2.2 Developmental Profile II (Alpern, Bol and Shearer, 1986)

This indirect test, administered by a psychologist as a semi-structured interview with a caregiver of a child, is suitable for the period of birth to 9 years 6 months. There are five scales covering five functional domains required for the present study. The test was standardised on non-disabled children and the norms are based on parental report of the children's abilities. Each scale contains a list of items describing particular behaviours, arranged and weighted according to the development of non-disabled children. A child 'passes' or 'fails' on the items depending on whether the caregiver says the child can or cannot exhibit the behaviour described. The total number of items 'passed' can yield a criterion-referenced raw score, while the sum of weights attached to each item 'passed' yields a norm-referenced developmental age in months. Subtracting chronological age from developmental age yields an age-differential.

The following is a listing of the scales and the range of functions that each raw score can reflect. Items within a scale vary greatly and the range of functions bearing on a raw score depends on the particular mixture of items passed. Hence, children receiving similar raw scores may not be qualitatively similar in functioning.

6.2.2.1 Academic

This scale assesses such skills as whether a child has a concept of size, number and time; whether there is an understanding of the association between spoken words and colours, objects and pictures; whether a range of paper-and-pencil skills can be performed; academic achievement. There are 34 items of the following type: responds to others, responds to objects, has likes and dislikes, searches for something hidden, marks paper, knows body parts, associates word to object/picture, recognises self, categorises, copies lines, concept of size, concept of number, copies circles, names colours, copies/draws square, rhymes words, copies/draws triangles, names objects, knows own address, recalls story content, promoted through grades, prints and writes, knows days of week, multiples, remembers telephone numbers/addresses (raw score range 0 to 34). The sum of weights attached to each item, which yields a developmental age in months, can be used to calculate an IQ.

6.2.2.2 Communication

This scale has items related to the ability to understand language, communicate non-verbally, communicate verbally and to control elements of speech and articulation. There are 38 items of the following type: 'plays' with vocal noises, has babble 'speech', responds to sounds, imitates words, communicates non-verbally, communicates verbally, names objects, carries out commands, uses 15 words correctly, communicate 'more'/'another', uses short sentences, repeats parts of rhymes, names pictures, uses 50 words, says own name, says/sings rhymes, knows own sex, tells story from pictures, talks on telephone, purchases, says own age, seeks meaning of words, tells story without pictures, uses argument, recognises written words, dials number, recites pledge, reads aloud, retells plot, understands non-verbal gestures, rhymes words, follows radio programme, writes letter (raw score range 0 to 38).

6.2.2.3   Physical

Items in this scale are concerned with gross-motor abilities such as posture control, mobility and locomotion; fine-motor abilities involving movement of the hands and fingers; control of the facial muscles. The 39 items are of the following type: lies down and holds up head, rolls, creeps/crawls, opposes finger to thumb, crawls-sits-stands, does not drool, uses stairs, walks avoiding objects, unwraps objects, throws, uses tricycle, copies line, jumps up and down, leaps forward, cuts out, hops, uses door latch/knob, catches, jumps rope, uses key, makes snowball and throws, plays hop-scotch, uses rollerskates/skateboard/iceskates, runs while carrying something, catches with one hand, uses matches, winks, whistles, plays sports, uses bicycle (raw score range 0 to 39).

6.2.2.4   Social

This scale is concerned with personal and interpersonal behaviours that reflect social competence. There are 36 items of the following type: wants attention, babble talks, shows negative reactions, waves, has concept of 'my', responds to instructions, keeps self busy and content, shows interest in other children's activities, shows jealousy, plays with breakable toy, explores new places, knows own and others sex, helps parents, indicates need for toilet, follows rules in group games, takes turns, uses toys appropriately, plays with one other, understands ownership by others, draws a man, plays in neighbourhood, says please and thankyou, has interest in own body parts, has knowledge of other's emotions and feelings, keeps secrets, plays table game, does home chores, knows about voting, plays make-believe, visits outside neighbourhood, purchases articles for others (raw score range 0 to 36).

6.2.2.5   Self-Help

This scale assesses skills related to self-care behaviour and independence in activities of daily living. The 39 items are of the following type: gets out-of-reach objects, grasps and holds, holds bottle while drinking, helps with dressing, drinks from cup/glass, gets about house without being watched, takes off footwear, knows difference between edible and non-edible, takes off coat, dries hands, understands dangers, puts on coat, undoes buttons/laces/zippers, puts on shoes, cares for toilet needs, toilet trained, washes/dries face and hands, dresses completely, puts away toys, answers telephone correctly, brushes/combs hair, does household chores, builds or mends, bathes and dries, uses cutlery, decides on clothes to wear, purchases, prepares food, cares for animals (raw score range 0 to 39).

6.2.3   Pictorial Test of Intelligence (French, 1964)

This direct test, administered by a psychologist, was designed and has been found suitable for non-disabled and disabled children (Coop, Eckel and Stuck, 1975; McCarty et al, 1986) between three and eight years of age. General cognitive ability may be relevant to the effectiveness of various types of intervention in cerebral palsy (Goldkamp, 1984; Parette and Hourcade, 1984). This test has six scales covering a range of functions within the cognitive domain. One scale is related in content to Achievement Tests to be described (Section 6.2.4) while another is related to the language assessment domain (Section 6.2.5). The test was standardised on non-disabled children but the instructions, materials and multiple choice format permit physically and verbally disabled children to respond merely by looking at their choice. Questions, generally, are presented orally by the examiner while the child is shown large picture cards on which are presented four possible choices or answers. Each scale yields a criterion-referenced raw score based on the number of correct responses and the raw scores can be converted to norm-referenced mental age equivalents by reference to tables. The total score for the six scales can be converted to an overall mental age and IQ.

6.2.3.1   Immediate Recall

This has 19 items and measures the ability to retain and recall visual patterns. A stimulus card is presented for five seconds and then removed from view. A multiple choice response card is immediately shown for the child to identify the same drawing (raw score range 0 to 19).

6.2.3.2   Form Discrimination

This has 27 items and measures the ability to visually match forms and to visually discriminate between similar shapes. The child is required to match a drawing on a stimulus card with one of four drawings on a response card (raw score range 0 to 27).

6.2.3.3   Similarities

Three drawings on each response card possess common elements while one drawing does not belong to the set. The child's task is to determine the three drawings that 'go together' and recognise the one drawing that does not 'belong' with the others. The common elements in three of the four drawings must be perceived and brought together into a single concept. Responses reveal the child's ability to generalize using visual information. There are 22 items (raw score range 0 to 22).

6.2.3.4 Information and Comprehension

This is designed to sample a range of knowledge and general understanding. It includes questions relating to the use of objects, properties of objects, origins of things, the association between colours and names, and the association between pictures and names. There are 29 items (raw score range 0 to 29).

6.2.3.5 Size and Number

Perception and recognition of size, number symbol recognition and comprehension, ability to solve simple arithmetic problems and telling the time are sampled by this scale. Some of the 31 items are related in content to the Achievement Tests described in Section 6.2.4 (raw score range 0 to 31).

6.2.3.6 Picture Vocabulary

This has 32 items and assesses verbal comprehension and requires recall of previously acquired verbal meanings in the association of pictures to spoken words. A child must respond to a word spoken by the examiner and select one of four drawings which best represents the meaning of the spoken word. The scale is therefore related in content to the language assessment domain described in Section 6.2.5 (raw score range 0 to 32).

6.2.3.7 General Cognition

The total raw score for the above six scales gives a global measure of general cognitive ability embracing all the above functions (raw score range 0 to 160).

6.2.4 Achievement Test

The direct tests in this section, administered by a psychologist, were designed for the present project as assessments of academic achievement. They are related in content to parts of Developmental Profile II (Section 6.6.2) and Pictorial Test of Intelligence (Section 6.2.3) and attainment records have been shown to be correlated to other Developmental indices (Krasner and Silverstein, 1976). Various educationalists were consulted during the design of the tests. Some items have been adapted from other standardised and non-standardised tests. Instructions, materials and multiple-choice formats permit physically and verbally disabled children with cerebral palsy to respond and demonstrate their academic skills. Each item is scored 0 or 1 depending on whether the child's response is incorrect or correct and the total number of items passed yield criterion-referenced raw scores. The tests have not been normed.

6.2.4.1 Reading

A pre-reading selection with three parts is designed to measure pre-requisite skills for reading and spelling while a formal reading section with two parts assesses sight vocabulary and comprehension of printed words and grammar (raw score total range 0 to 82).

6.2.4.1.1 Pre-Reading

Visual sequential memory. The child is shown cards with two or three item sequences of pictures, shapes, letters and words. A given sequence is shown for five seconds and then removed. The child is then shown another card with either two or three alternative sequences and must choose the 'correct' sequence. There are eight items; two sequences each of pictures, shapes, letters and words (raw score range 0 to 8).

Individual letter recognition. The child is shown a card with the 26 letters of the alphabet in lower-case. The test pronounces the letters in a predetermined random order and the child must indicate the correct symbol for the given sound (raw score range 0 to 26).

Recognition of upper-case and lower-case pairs of letters. A card is shown with three pairs of letters, one pair correct and two pairs incorrect. The child must indicate the correct pair. There are 13 items of varying difficulty (raw score range 0 to 13).

6.2.4.1.2 Formal Reading

Phonetically regular printed word recognition. The child is required to indicate a printed word associated with a word spoken by the tester. A card is shown with 15 printed words. Each word has two or three letters. The tester reads the words in a predetermined order and the child must indicate the correct printed word (raw score range 0 to 15).

Comprehension of printed words and grammar. A card is shown with an incomplete sentence. Five printed words are provided as alternatives for the child to complete the sentence. The tester does not read the sentence or the words, but has established with practice items that the child must select the correct word to complete the sentence. There are 20 items (raw score range 0 to 20).

6.2.4.2 Mathematics

A number section with two parts is designed to measure the concept of number and recognition of number symbols, a measurement section is concerned with knowledge of length, height, width, size, weight and volume and a third section is concerned with arithmetic operators (raw score total, range 0 to 66).

6.2.4.2.1 *Number*

Number concept. For each of 10 items a card is shown on which is printed a number of objects. The child must indicate how many printed objects there are (raw score range 0 to 10).

Number symbol recognition. For each of 15 items, a card is shown with printed number symbols. The tester asks the child to indicate particular numbers (raw score range 0 to 15).

6.2.4.2.2 *Measurement*

The child is shown items of varying height, length, width, and size, is provided with boxes of different weight, and is shown a card with printed jugs containing various amounts of liquid. The child has to respond to questions (number of questions in brackets) concerning height (3), length (1), width (3), size (3), weight (4), and volume (6) (raw score range 0 to 20).

6.2.4.2.3 *Arithmetic Operators*

There are 10 items concerned with addition and subtraction. For each item a card is shown with a number of printed objects. The tester tells the child how many there are, and asks the child, who must then indicate, how many there would be if a given number were put with, or taken away from, those present. There are six items concerned with the formal operation of 'plus' and 'minus'. For each item a card is shown with two numbers and an operator. The child must select the correct answer from four printed number symbols. There are three items concerned with the foundation of multiplication; questions deal with repeated addition. There are three items concerned with the foundation of division; questions deal with sharing in an imaginary situation (raw score range 0 to 22).

6.2.5 Language Assessment

This assessment, assembled and administered by a speech therapist, is made up mostly of direct tests and includes an assessment of the vocal apparatus, pre-verbal communication, articulation and expressive language. A number of published tests are used and some of these have been normed which allows for the collection of norm-referenced data. Other parts of the assessment have been derived from published tests and yield criterion-referenced data only. All direct testing is routinely video-recorded, yielding a record of all verbal and non-verbal communication taking place during a testing session. Many of the performance measures are taken from the video recordings rather than while testing, allowing for the greatest possible freedom of communication between therapist and child. Parts of the assessment are related in content to parts of Developmental Profile II (Section 6.2.2) and Pictorial Test of Intelligence (Section 6.2.3).

6.2.5.1 Dysarthria Assessment

This direct assessment is based largely on items from the Frenchay Dysarthria Assessment (Enderby, 1983) but also on the Fletcher Time-by-Count Test of Diadochokinetic Syllable Rate (1978) and yields criterion-referenced data only.

6.2.5.1.1 *Motor Control 1 (raw score total, range 16 to 128)*

Control of the speech mechanism in the absence of sound. For the following seven items, performance is scored on a scale of 1 (maximum abnormality) to 5 (no difficulty/abnormality); coughing, swallowing, dribbling, lips at rest, lips spread, jaw at rest, palate in eating. For an eighth item the child is required to imitate the following four actions; put tongue out, move tongue in and out, move tongue up and down, move tongue side to side. For each part, a rating of 0 (unrecognisable response or no response), 1 (incomplete movement) or 2 (accurate movement) is given (raw score range 7 to 43).

Control of the speech mechanisms when sounds are produced. For the following nine items, performance is rated on a scale of 1 (maximum abnormality) to 5 (no difficulty/abnormality); respiration in speech, lips in speech, jaw in speech, palate in speech, pitch, volume, prosody, tongue in speech, intelligibility. A tenth item requires the child to produce the following 10 sounds in isolation after demonstration by the tester; 'a', 'i', 'u', 'm', 'p', 't', 'k', 'f', 'l', 's'. An eleventh item requires the production of the following five syllable strings: 'kala', 'pata, paka', 'taka', 'pataka'. The twelfth item requires the rapid repetition of the following five consonants; 'p', 't', 'k', 'f', 'l'. Each part of the above three items is given a rating of 0 (unrecognisable response), 1 (inaccurate response) or 2 (accurate articulation) according to set criteria (raw score range 9 to 85).

6.2.5.1.2 *Motor Control 2*

The child is required to make 20 repetitions of the following sounds; 'p', 't', 'k', 'f', 'l'. The tester uses pictures which represent the sounds in order to assist the child. The time taken to make 20 repetitions is recorded, and the rate of repetition (sounds/sec) calculated. If the child cannot make 20 repetitions of a sound, a rate of 0 is recorded. The mean repetition rate for the five sounds is calculated (raw score range 0 to maximum rate).

6.2.5.2 Pre-Verbal Communication

This assessment is a significant re-working of a schedule devised by Kiernan and Reid (1987). Most items involve indirect assessment and the parent is asked whether particular capacities or behaviours are demonstrated by the child. A few items involve direct testing. The original schedule has three scoring formats; 'never, rarely, usually', 'no-yes', 'number of times the child makes the correct response out of a given number of presentations'. A single system of scoring was required for the present study in which higher numbers are associated with more desirable forms of communication. Some items from the schedule have been dropped because they are unscorable in terms of desirability. As a rule, the 'never, rarely, usually' format is converted to '0, 1, 2'. A higher score of '3' is awarded if the child has developed beyond the need to show the capacity or behaviour described in the item, or has a more advanced non-verbal system of communication, or uses speech. Behaviours described by some items cannot be supplanted by a superior form of behaviour, in which case '2' is the highest score possible. All data are criterion-referenced only.

6.2.5.2.1 Motor Control 3

All 13 items in the 'vocal imitation' section are used some of which involve direct testing while others depend on parent and teacher report: i. makes non-speech noises in response to speech by another person; ii. makes speech noises when talked to; iii. clearly initiates speech sounds made by adults; iv. will blow through lips when you do (blow a 'raspberry'); v. will imitate a cough; vi. imitates own sounds when played on a tape recorder; vii. imitates the pleasure sounds of other children; viii. imitates animal noises which you make; ix. imitates words when they are spoken but does not necessarily use words for communication; x. imitates the distress sounds of other children; ix. imitates voice intonation patterns of other children; xii. will show clear imitation of words but only after a delay; xiii. will imitate words when the word or phrase is said by other person and will imitate with a delay of five minutes or more, but not necessarily for communication. Items iv, v, vii, viii and x are not scored '3' because they cannot be surplanted by a superior form of verbal behaviour (raw score range 0 to 34).

6.2.5.2.2 Receptive Non-Verbal

All eight items of the 'understanding non-vocal communication' section are used some of which involve direct testing while others depend on parent and teacher report: i. takes a neutral object from another person when it is offered; ii. takes another person's hand when it is held out; iii. looks to where another person is pointing when the other person has a finger on the object; iv. looks at an object to which the person is pointing when the object is within two metres from the person who is pointing; v. cooperates when being physically guided (prompted) and then repeats desired action independently; vi. looks at where the other person is pointing when the object is more distant than two metres from the person who is pointing; vii. follows simple direction when gestures are used with or without speech; viii. the child's attention can be directed to an object by looking at the child and then the object repeatedly, without pointing. In the original schedule these items are scored as the number of times the child makes the correct response out of three presentations. This scoring system is retained and the child receives a score of 0, 1, 2 or 3 if demonstrating the behaviour 0, 1, 2, or 3 times out of 3, respectively (raw score range 0 to 24).

6.2.5.2.3 *Expressive Non-Verbal*

Six sections of the original schedule are all related to non-verbal communication (raw score range 0 to 83).

Attention Seeking. Four of the original five items are used: i. reaches out to be lifted or hugged; ii. approaches and touches another person to get attention; iii. approaches another person and makes sounds to get attention; iv. approaches another person and vocalizes to get attention. Item i is not scored 3 because the behaviour should persist even after the child can speak. The following item from the original schedule was dropped because it is unscorable in terms of desirability: cries, the crying being directed at another person (raw score range 0 to 11).

Need Satisfaction. All eight of the original items are used: i. points to a picture or object to indicate preference or need; ii. gives another person an object related to the solution of a problem the child wants the other person to solve; iii. looks for a picture of an object to represent a need; iv. uses a simple gesture to indicate needs; v. pushes or pulls another person to induce them to go somewhere or get something that the child needs; vi. touches an object the child wants and then glances at the other person and object alternately until the other person responds; vii. points with hand and/or arm to distant object the child wants whilst looking alternately at the other person and the object; viii. smiles when the child wants something, as equivalent to 'can I have?' (raw score range 0 to 24).

Simple Negation. Three of the original five items are used: i. waves goodbye to indicate she wants another person to go away; ii. pushes another person's hand away when the child does not want help; iii. frowns at another person to express displeasure or questioning. The following items are not included because they are unscorable in terms of desirability: will go limp or lie on the floor to resist; hits another person when they frustrate the child (raw scores range 0 to 9).

Positive Interaction. Five of the original six items are used: i. shows an object to another person spontaneously and gives it if requested; ii. gives object to other people without being asked and without them necessarily wanting the objects; iii. waves goodbye without prompting when another person is leaving or when the child is leaving; iv. will have one-to-one 'conversation' with another person; v. kisses or hugs other people as an expression of affection. Item v is not scored 3 since such behaviour should persist even when the child has speech. The following item is not included because it is unscorable in terms of desirability: smiles or hugs another person who is irritated with the child in order to placate them (raw score range 0 to 14).

Shared Attention. All five of the original items are used: i. shows a picture of an object only to draw attention to the object; ii. shows an object only to draw attention to another object; iii. pushes or pulls another person only to show them something or someone; iv. points with hand and/or arm to distant objects to draw attention to them; v. vocalises simply to draw attention to an object, equivalent to 'look, there it is' (raw score range 0 to 15).

Spontaneous Use of Symbols or Signs: a score of 0, 1, 2, 3, 4, 5, 6, 7, 8, 9, 10 is given if the child uses 0, 1, 2, 3, 4, 5–7, 8–10, 11–13, 14–20, 21–50, more than 50, symbols or signs spontaneously for communication. A score of 10 is also given if the child's speech is sufficiently adequate not to require the use of symbols or signs (raw score range 0 to 10).

6.2.5.2.4 *Receptive Verbal*

Thirteen of the original 14 items of the 'understanding of vocalisation and speech' section are used: i. responds to own name, as opposed to names of other children, when own name spoken; ii. stops activity when told 'no' or 'stop'; iii. hands to the tester, or points to, six or more different familiar objects which are laid out in front of the child when asked to 'show me . . .' or 'give me . . .'; iv. responds to simple spoken request without gestures, eg., 'come here', 'sit down'; v. points to parts of child's own body on request; vi. follows simple directions like 'get your coat', 'close the door', without gestures or strong cues; vii. points to or goes to four or five familiar people on request; viii. shows four or five pictures when requested; ix. responds appropriately to questions like 'where is your bag', when objects are not in view; x. follows spoken directions like 'put spoon in the cup' where there is an action and two objects; xi. points to or goes to four or five places in the home, school or centre on request; xii. understands sentences with adjectives, eg. 'give me the little ball'; xiii. understands instructions containing words like 'on', 'in' and 'under' without gestures. The following item from the original schedule is not included because it is unscorable in terms of desirability; will put hands over ears if the child does not want to do what she is asked. The maximum score for all items is 2 (raw score range 0 to 26).

6.2.5.3 Articulation

The Edinburgh Articulation Test (Anthony et al, 1971) is used for this part of the assessment. It is a direct test which assesses the ability to articulate consonants. The child is presented with a series of pictures and asked to name them. The intention is for the child to concentrate on the materials presented, rather than on the pronunciation of a word. The aim is to elicit, as far as possible, spontaneous utterances by the presentation of the pictures. The articulation of consonants in words uttered in isolation is assessed; no attention is given to vowels, and no attention is given to rhythm or intonation. The test has 68 items each of which is scored 0 (fail) or 1 (pass). It has been normed on non-disabled children aged between three years and up to six years. Six years is considered to be the terminal stage for the development of articulation in non-disabled children although children who are disabled can be much older before reaching the raw score ceiling. The criterion-referenced raw score total can be converted to a norm-referenced standard score and an age equivalent by reference to a table. The table is very difficult to use, and conversion rules had to be set for the present project (raw score range 0 to 68).

6.2.5.4   Expressive Verbal

The Expressive Language Scale of the Reynell Developmental Language Scales (Reynell, 1985) is used for this assessment. This is a direct test with three sections.

Language Structure. This section assesses language from the earliest stages of pre-language, and covers language structure from the earliest vocalisation to the use of complex sentences with subordinate clauses. It is concerned with spontaneous expression, and is scored incidentally during the course of an interview with the child. In the present project, the tester talked to each child in the classroom situation. The child was then withdrawn for the assessment which was video-recorded and began with 15 minutes of one-to-one play and conversation with the tester. Language was sometimes spontaneous and sometimes elicited by the tester during this 'conversation session', the purpose of which was to establish a relationship and rapport between the tester and the child. There followed a more formal interview with the child. All sounds, words and sentences uttered by the child before, during and after the period of this phase of the assessment were documented and the video-recordings were replayed for this purpose. The section was scored last after all other phases of the assessment were completed.

Vocabulary. The child is questioned about objects and pictures, and scored according to any verbal responses. The child is also asked questions when no object or picture is present (eg, 'what is an apple?') which tests the ability to describe an internalised concept. The items are presented and scored according to the manual. The items are ordered in increasing difficulty, but are said to be within the experience of even housebound disabled children.

Language Content. This section assesses the creative uses of language. The child is asked to describe a picture. All ideas must come from the child, and the aim is to find out how far language is used creatively in describing the picture. To succeed, the child must be able to verbalise connected thoughts. The section is scored according to the manual, and articulatory errors are not penalised. While all responses made by children are not explicitly mentioned in the manual, the criteria for scoring, in practice, cover most responses. For the present project, rules were established to cover ambiguous responses.

The assessment yields criterion-referenced raw scores for the three sections and a raw score total (raw score range 0 to 67). The scale has been normed on non-disabled children aged between 1.5 and 7 years which is the important period for normal language development. Children with disabilities can, however, be much older than 7 years before reaching the raw score ceiling. The total raw score can be converted to a norm-referenced standard score and age equivalent by referring to tables.

6.2.6 Fine-Motor Assessment

The direct tests in this section, administered by a psychologist, were designed for the present project because previously published tests (eg., Jarvis and Hey, 1984; Reddihough et al, 1990) were not suitable. Some items resemble clinical tests used in developmental paediatrics, tests used in occupational therapy assessments, and items in the Perceptual-Motor Abilities Test (Laszlo and Bairstow, 1985). The tasks, in the order in which they are given, are as follows: using pen and paper, transferring pegs on a pegboard, building a tower of blocks, transferring balls between trays, manipulating a nut on a threaded rod, threading beads. The hand used by the child to perform the pen and paper tasks is designed the 'preferred-hand'. All tasks are first demonstrated by the tester. The tester assists the child when attempting a task, but only the minimum assistance is given to enable the child to complete the task. Performance is video-recorded with 0.1 sec time base with cameras focused on the hands and arms of the child. Criterion-referenced scores are taken from the video recordings according to written criteria. The assessment has not been normed. Data from the tower-of-blocks task and a free drawing task are not considered in this report. Parts of the assessment are related in content to Developmental Profile II (Section 6.2.2).

6.2.6.1 Fine-Motor Independence

The full assessment requires the following twelve activities; transferring pegs on a pegboard with the (i) preferred and (ii) nonpreferred-hand, transferring balls between trays with the (iii) preferred and (iv) nonpreferred-hand, manipulating a nut (v) upwards and (vi) downwards, (vii) using two hands cooperatively to thread beads onto a string, (viii) accurately placing pen on paper, tracing between (ix) horizontal and (x) vertical lines, tracing over (xi) horizontal and (xii) vertical lines. The independence of the child in carrying out each of these activities is scored from the video-recordings as follows; 3 if no physical assistance is given, 2 if some physical assistance is given but it is unclear whether it was essential, 1 if assistance was given and the child could not have done the task without assistance, 0 if the child could not actively participate in the task or if the task was not attempted. The sum of scores for the twelve activities is a global measure of the degree of independence in carrying out a range of different tasks with the hands (raw score range 0 to 36).

6.2.6.2   Object Transfer 1

Two tasks in the assessment require the child to grasp, transfer and place five pegs on a pegboard first with the (i) preferred-hand and then with the (ii) nonpreferred-hand. The five pegs, each 8.0 cm long and 1.8 cm in diameter are placed in line in a five × five hole pegboard. The task is to transfer the five pegs in a particular order from the penultimate distant line of holes, to the nearest line of holes. The child is encouraged to complete the task as rapidly as possible. Only one measure of performance is used. In each task, the number of pegs transferred is divided by the time taken to perform the task to obtain the 'rate of transfer'. If no pegs are transferred, the rate of transfer is 0. The mean rate of transfer for the two tasks (pegs/sec) gives an overall measure of ability to reach and grasp an object which is physically constrained and to place and release the object under similarly constrained conditions. Using the mean of performance of the two hands, get around the problems of deciding which hand is the 'preferred-hand' in those few children who do not seem to have a marked hand preference (raw score range 0 to maximum rate of transfer).

6.2.6.3   Object Transfer 2

Two tasks require the child to grasp, transfer and release five pairs of balls of various size and weight between two trays first with the (i) preferred-hand and then with the (ii) nonpreferred-hand. The five pairs of balls of sizes varying from a pair of cricket balls (7.0 cm diameter), through a pair of golf balls (4.1 cm diameter), down to a pair of small marbles (1.6 cm diameter), are placed in a circular dish 24 cm diameter and 5.5 cm deep. The tray is tilted slightly towards the subject so the balls collect at the near side. The task is to transfer the balls, in any order, to another dish of similar dimensions placed immediately adjacent. The child is encouraged to complete the task as rapidly as possible. Only one measure of performance is used. In each task, the number of balls transferred is divided by the time taken to perform the task to obtain the 'rate of transfer'. If no balls are transferred the rate of transfer is 0. The mean rate of transfer for the two tasks (ball/sec) gives an overall measure of ability to reach and grasp objects which are minimally constrained and to place and release the objects under similarly unconstrained conditions (raw score range 0 to maximum rate of transfer).

6.2.6.4   Manipulation

Two tasks require the child to manipulate a plastic nut along a threaded plastic rod by first screwing it (i) downwards and then screwing it (ii) upwards. The threaded rod, 13.5cm long and 4.0cm diameter and mounted vertically on a base plate, is placed before the child. A plastic nut (7.0cm in diameter) is placed at the top of the rod, and the task is to manipulate the nut with either hand, and screw it down the rod as rapidly as possible. Similarly, a plastic nut is placed at the bottom of the rod, and the task is to manipulate it with either hand and screw it upwards. In each case the vertical distance moved by the nut is divided by the time taken to obtain the 'rate of manipulation'. If the nut cannot be moved along the rod, the rate of movement is 0. The mean rate of movement (mm/sec) gives an overall measure of ability to manipulate an object with the hand (raw score range 0 to maximum rate).

6.2.6.5   Two-Hand Coordination

One task requires five beads to be threaded onto a piece of string. The five beads 3.5cm in diameter, each pierced by a hole 0.9cm diameter, are made available, one at a time, to the child. A piece of string 70.0cm long, with the end 1.3cm stiffened, is also made available. The task is to thread the beads onto the string. The task is complex, requiring gripping a bead in one hand with the hole orientated appropriately, while holding the pliable string in the other hand with at least 5.0cm free to push through the hole. The string then has to be released so the hand that was holding it, can now grasp the bead. The hand that was holding the bead should then release it, and grasp the string to pull it through the hole. Hence, both hands are involved in grasping and releasing actions (grasping and releasing the bead, and grasping and releasing the string) and both hands are involved in accurate aiming and placement. All of these elements are found in the tasks described previously, but this task has the additional difficulty of requiring the hands to be controlled cooperatively. The number of beads threaded is divided by the time taken to obtain the 'rate of coordination'. If no beads are threaded the rate of coordination is 0 (raw score range 0 to maximum rate).

6.2.6.6   Pen Placement

One task requires the accurate placement of a pen on eleven 0.1cm dots printed on a piece of paper in an inverted 'V' configuration (20.0cm high, 15.0cm wide at the base). The task is to mark each dot with the pen precisely, alternating between dots on each 'wing' of the inverted 'V'; increasingly larger amplitudes of movement are therefore required for each accurate placement of the pen as the child moves down the paper. The child is therefore required to hold a pen in a way appropriate for marking paper and to accurately aim the pen at the set of targets. Only one measure of performance will be used. The closest distance between each mark and the printed dots is measured in mm and the mean is calculated. If no mark is made on the paper an arbitrary value of 305mm is given which is the largest distance between a printed dot and the edge of the paper. The score gives a measure of ability to mark paper accurately with a pen. The measure of error is multiplied by −1 so that large scores indicate good performance (raw score range −305mm to 0mm).

6.2.6.7 Drawing

There are four tasks requiring the following; tracing between pairs of parallel (i) vertical and (ii) horizontal printed lines 0.3cm apart and 8.0cm long, tracing over a (iii) vertical and (iv) horizontal printed line 8.0cm long. The child is therefore required to hold a pen in a way appropriate for marking paper and to accurately guide the pen in relation to boundaries. Only one measure of performance will be used. In each task the measure of error is a form of integrated absolute error which encompasses errors in the overall orientation and straightness of the child's mark but not errors in placement. If the child does not mark the paper an arbitrary error value of 205mm is given which is the largest distance between the printed lines and the edge of the paper. The mean error for the four tasks gives a global measure of ability to draw straight lines given boundaries to guide the movement. The measure of error is multiplied by −1 so that large scores indicate good performance (raw score range −205mm to 0mm).

6.2.7 Gross-Motor Assessment

The direct tests in this section, administered by a psychologist and a physiotherapist, were designed for the present project. Some items resemble clinical tests used in developmental paediatrics (Holt, 1981) and tests in physiotherapy assessments. The assessments at the beginning of the study were carried out in a hospital unit which incorporated a laboratory for the assessment of gait, because the intention was to develop a gait analysis methodolgy suitable for the type of young child with limited ability to ambulate, who was to be included in the study. Although the value of gait analysis in cerebral palsy is recognised (Deluca, 1991; Gage, 1983; Patrick, 1989; Winters and Gage, 1985) there was insufficient time to establish a suitable methodolgy and the use of the laboratory's facilities extended only to the video-cameras. Since Video-recordings could just as easily be done elsewhere, assessments at the end of the study were carried out in the particular institution in which a child was enrolled, using portable video-cameras. Each child attempted a sequence of 18 tasks. Shoes were removed, no physical aids were given (eg. no splints, crutches, etc) and the physiotherapist gave only the minimum assistance necessary for performance of an activity. All criterion-referenced timed scores were taken from the video-recordings according to written criteria. It has been found that gait velocity is a good single indicator of gait ability (Larsson et al, 1986; Norlin and Odenrick, 1986) and the general principle employed in the present assessment was that the more able the child the longer would a static position be maintained, the faster would a postural change be carried out and the higher the speed of ambulation.

Before an assessment was carried out, a parent was interviewed and asked whether the child will be able to perform each of the 18 tasks and an estimated 'independence score' of the following general form was given; 0 if the child will not be able to contribute actively to performance of the task even with assistance, 1 if the child will require assistance from the therapist, 3 if the parent estimates that the child will be able to complete the task without assistance. If assistance is needed, the parent is asked to describe the type of assistance. At the end of the study, staff involved with the education of the children were interviewed rather than the parent. The purpose of the interview was twofold; to give the therapist information in advance as a guide to what kind of assistance might be required, to check whether the child's performance in the test situation is representative of everyday performance with which the parent is familiar.

Each of the 18 tasks is given a second 'independence score' when the video-recordings are replayed for the purpose of obtaining timed scores: 0 if performance does not satisfy the written criteria for the task or the therapist was entirely responsible for any apparent performance by the child, with the child not actively engaged in the task, or if the task was not attempted; 1 if performance satisfies the written criteria for the task and the therapist gave assistance which was essential for the child and the child is actively engaged in carrying out the task; 2 if performance satisfies the written criteria for the task but the therapist physically intervened to assist the child and it is unclear whether the intervention was actually essential for the child to carry out and complete the task; 3 if performance satisfies the written criteria for the task and the child required no physical assistance.

The following is a listing of the tasks together with a brief description of the timed measures which were taken from the video-recordings:

i. Sitting on a Stool. The child is required to sit on a stool with both hands on the knees, both feet on the floor (or on a box appropriate to the size of the child), with back and head held as erect as possible. The child is requested to remain still, and maintain the posture for 30sec. The measure of performance is how long the child manages to maintain the posture up to a maximum of 30sec.

ii. Sitting on the stool to sitting on the floor. The child is required to get down off the stool, onto the floor, and into a sitting posture. Any means of getting onto the floor is allowed and any mode of sitting on the floor is allowed. The duration of the activity is recorded. The height of the stool is 23cm. The child therefore moves vertically through a nett 23cm from start to finish. This constant is divided by the duration to obtain an estimate of 'rate of sitting'.

iii. Sitting on the floor in the child's preferred posture. If not already in the preferred sitting posture (as indicated by the parent), the child is asked to adopt it, and is given assistance if necessary. An instruction is given to sit as erect and as still as possible, and the length of the time the child can maintain the posture is measured up to a maximum of 30sec.

iv. Sitting on the floor to lying supine on the floor. The child is then instructed to lie down on the floor. Any mode of lying down is allowed. The length of time required to reach a supine posture is measured. The angle between the thigh and the trunk can be expected to increase by a nett 90 degrees from start to finish. This constant is divided by the duration to obtain an estimate of 'rate of lying'.

v. Lying supine on the floor. The child is instructed to lie flat and straight on the floor, with legs together and arms down at the side. The measure of performance is how long the child can maintain the posture, up to a maximum of 30sec.

vi. Full roll to the right. The child is required to roll to the right into the prone position, and to continue the action on into the supine position. The length of time required to complete the action is measured. The longitudinal axis of the child moves through a nett 360 degrees from start to finish. This constant is divided by the duration to obtain an estimate of 'rate of rolling'.

vii. Full roll to the left. This phase is the same as above, but in reverse.

viii. Lying prone. The child is asked to roll into the prone position, and lie flat and straight with legs together and arms down at the side. The measure of performance is how long the child can maintain the posture, up to a maximum of 30sec.

ix. Lying prone to four point kneeling. The time required for the child to move from the prone position to a four point kneeling posture is measured. The angle between the upper arm and the trunk can be expected to increase by a nett 90 degrees from start to finish. This constant is divided by the duration to obtain an estimate of 'rate of kneeling'.

x. Four point kneeling. The child is required to maintain a four point kneeling posture, with head free of the floor, elbows extended, hands in contact with the floor, partial weight bearing through the arms, back parallel with the floor, knees in contact with the floor and partial weight bearing through the knees. The length of time the child can maintain the posture is measured, up to a maximum of 30sec.

xi. Crawling. A distance of 225cm is marked on the floor with tapes, and the child is required to crawl the distance between the tapes. The action required is for the trunk to be free of the floor and parallel to the floor, weight bearing through the hands and knees, arms and legs moving reciprocally and alternately. If this action is not possible independent of the therapist, crawling with assistance is not attempted because there is no satisfactory way for the therapist to support the child and assist with double reciprocal movements of arms and legs. The time taken to perform the task is measured. The distance moved is divided by the duration to obtain an estimate of 'rate of crawling'.

xii. Four point kneeling to high kneeling.   The time required for the child to move from a four point kneeling posture to a high kneeling posture is measured. The angle between the thigh and the trunk can be expected to increase by a nett 90 degrees from start to finish. This constant is divided by the duration to obtain an estimate of 'rate of kneeling'.

xiii. High kneeling.   The child is required to maintain a high kneeling posture defined as follows; head and trunk upright, hips extended with thighs in-line with the trunk, lower legs at right angles with the thighs, weight bearing through the knees, hands and arms free of the floor. The length of time up to a maximum of 30sec is measured.

xiv. High kneeling to standing.   Movement between a high kneeling posture to a standing posture is required, and the time required for carrying out the action is measured. The angle between the upper and lower leg can be expected to increase by a nett 90 degrees from start to finish. This constant is divided by the duration to obtain an estimate of 'rate of standing'.

NB: Some cerebral palsied children find kneeling, crawling and high kneeling impossible even with assistance. If it is clear that the child cannot be assisted through the above five tasks, they are not attempted.

xv. Standing.   The child is required to stand in one place, weight bearing through both feet, knees and hips extended, and with trunk and head erect for an interval up to 30sec duration.

xvi. Walking.   A distance of 225cm is marked on the floor with tapes, and the child is required to walk the distance between the tapes. A reciprocal stepping action is required with weight bearing through alternate legs and forward progression of the body. The child is discouraged from trotting or running. The time taken to perform the task is measured. The distance moved is divided by the duration to obtain an estimate of 'rate of walking'.

xvii. Standing to sitting on a stool.   The requirement here is for the child to stand with back to the stool, and to move from the standing posture to sitting on the stool. The time interval is measured. The angle between the thigh and the trunk can be expected to decrease by a nett 90 degrees from start to finish. This constant is divided by the duration to obtain an estimate of 'rate of sitting'.

xviii. 'Preferred' method of locomotion. The final phase requires the child to move the 225cm between the tapes on the floor, by whatever means is used ordinarily in the situation where there is no assistance, and no object or physical aid on which to rely. Any form of locomotion is allowed; eg, rolling, commando crawling, bottom shuffling, crawling on hands and knees, walking. This phase of the assessment is conducted as a 'race'. The time taken to perform the task is measured. The distance moved is divided by the duration to obtain an estimate of 'rate of locomotion'.

For all tasks requiring the maintenance of steady posture, if the child could not actively contribute anything toward maintenance of the posture, or if the posture could not be attempted, a duration of 0sec is recorded. For all tasks requiring mobility, if the child could not actively contribute anything toward the task, or if the task could not be attempted, a rate of 0degrees/sec or 0mm/sec is recorded.

In the following sections, task ii is included in Position Changing Independence (Section 6.2.7.2.) but not in Position Changing (Section 6.2.7.7) because of difficulties in defining the end point of the activity arising from the fact that many children cannot be assisted down from the stool directly into a seated posture. Task xvii is included in Position Changing Independence (Section 6.2.7.2) but not in Position Changing (Section 6.2.7.7) because many children lack control in letting themselves down and thereby flop on to the stool yielding a spuriously high measure. All tasks involving the maintenance of static postures are included in Postural Independence (Section 6.2.7.1) but no timed measures of these tasks are used because most children can maintain most postures up to a ceiling of 30sec when given assitance. Long durations, therefore, do not necessarily indicate good control.

6.2.7.1   Postural Independence

The sum of independence scores for the seven tasks requiring the maintenance of static postures (Section 6.2.7, i, iii, v, viii, x, xiii, xv) is a global measure of independence in maintaining postures (raw score range 0 to 21).

6.2.7.2   Position Changing Independence

The sum of independence scores for the eight tasks requiring movement from one posture to another posture (Section 6.2.7, ii, iv, vi, vii, ix, xii, xiv, xvii) is a global measure of independence in position changing (raw score range 0 to 24).

6.2.7.3   Crawling Independence

The independence score for task xi (Section 6.2.7) is a measure of independence in crawling (raw score range 0 to 3).

6.2.7.4   Walking Independence

The independence score for task xvi (Section 6.2.7) is a measure of independence in walking (raw score range 0 to 3).

6.2.7.5   Preferred Locomotion Independence

The independence score for task xviii (Section 6.2.7) is a measure of independence in locomotion (raw score range 0 to 3).

6.2.7.6   Locomotion Independence

The independence scores for tasks xi, xvi, and xviii are summed giving an overall measure of independence in locomotion (raw score range 0 to 9).

6.2.7.7   Position Changing

The mean rate for six of the eight position changing tasks (Section 6.2.7, iv, vi, vii, ix, xii, xiv) gives a global measure of ability to move from one posture to another (raw score range 0 to maximum rate).

6.2.7.8   Crawling

The rate of crawling in task xi (Section 6.2.7) is recorded (raw score range 0 to maximum rate).

6.2.7.9   Walking

The rate of walking in task xvi (Section 6.2.7) is recorded (raw score range 0 to maximum rate).

6.2.7.10   Preferred Locomotion

The rate of locomotion in task xviii (Section 6.2.7) is recorded (raw score range 0 to maximum rate).

6.2.8   Physical Assessment

A detailed physical and neurological examination is carrried out by a Consultant Orthopaedic Surgeon at the time of the Gross-Motor Assessment (Section 6.2.7) and is video-recorded. The parts of the examination used for the present study are described in the following sections.

6.2.8.1 Hip Mobility

There are 12 items (six each for the right and left limb) involving passive manipulation of the leg around the hip joint. The maximum amount of abduction, adduction, internal rotation, external rotation, and flexion is estimated in degrees according to a standard procedure. Normal angles (45, 35, 40, 45 and 120 degrees respectively) are subtracted from the obtained angles taking account of the sign; the larger the algebraic error the greater the amount of mobility in the hip joint. In addition, an estimate is made of any flexion deformity in the hip and the angle is given a −ve sign; the closer to zero the obtained angle, the less the amount of flexion deformity. The mean for the 12 items gives an overall index of hip mobility (raw score range, maximum −ve differential to positive differential indicating good mobility).

6.2.8.2 Hamstring Extensibility

There are four items (two each for the right and left leg) concerned with extensibility of the hamstring muscles. For 'straight leg raise' the difference between the normal angle of 80 degrees and the obtained angle is calculated taking account of the sign. For 'hamstring tightness' the obtained angle is given a negative sign. The mean of the four items gives an overall index of extensibility of the muscles on the dorsum of the leg and thigh (raw score range, maximum negative differential to positive differential indicating good mobility).

6.2.8.3 Height

A record is made of the height of the children (raw score is height in cm).

6.2.8.4 Weight

A record is kept of the weight of the children (raw score is weight in kg).

6.2.8.5 Neurological Assessment

The children are assessed for the presence or absence of postural reflex activity, and a prognosis is made of whether the children will eventually walk. The method described by Bleck (1975) is employed, and the following seven reflexes are tested; asymmetrical tonic neck reflex, symmetrical tonic neck reflex, Moro reflex, neck-righting reflex, foot placement reaction, parachute reaction, extensor thrust. For reflexes which are normally absent, the orthopaedic surgeon provides a score of '0' if the reflex is absent, '−0.5' if present but weak, '−1' if fully present. For reflexes which are normally present, the score is as follows; '0' if reflex is fully present, '−0.5' if present but weak, '−1' if absent. The total score for the seven reflexes is an index of abnormality. A total score of '0' indicates a good prognosis for walking, a total of '−1' is a guarded prognosis, while a total of '−2' or more is a poor prognosis for walking.

6.2.9   Adaptive Behaviour

This indirect assessment, administered by a psychologist, is termed 'adaptive behaviour' only because four of the five sections come from the Vineland Adaptive Behaviour Scales (Sparrow, Balla and Cicchetti, 1985). Adaptive behaviour is defined as performance of daily activities required for personal and social sufficiency. The scales are published in a number of forms including an Interview Edition covering ages between birth and 18 years 11 months and designed as a semi-structured interview for use with a parent or caregiver, and a Classroom Edition covering ages between 3 and 12 years 11 months and designed as a questionnaire to be completed by teachers. In the present study, three scales are taken from the Classroom Edition; namely, Personal Subdomain (here called Activities of Daily Living), Interpersonal Relationships Subdomain, and Play and Leisure Time Subdomain (here called Play). The fourth scale, namely Gross Motor Subdomain, is taken from the Interview Edition because the items start at lower ages and are more comprehensive than in the Classroom Edition and were therefore considered more appropriate for children with cerebral palsy in this study. Each scale is a check-list of items. Each item is scored 0, 1 or 2 depending on whether the behaviour described is never, sometimes or usually present in the child. The sum of scores yields a criterion-referenced raw score. The scales have been standardised on non-disabled children and the raw scores are converted to norm-referenced age equivalent scores by referring to tables.

The fifth scale, namely Attention and Control, was devised for the present study and is based on the 'Impulse Control' and 'Attention Span' behavioural stands in the Behavioural Characteristics Progression Observation Booklet (1973). This scale has not been normed and yields only a criterion-referenced score.

All five scales were administered as a semi-structured interview of a member of staff involved with the education of a child. The following is a listing of the scales and the range of functions that each raw score can reflect. The range of functions bearing on a raw score will depend on the particular mixture of items passed, hence, children receiving similar raw scores may not be qualitatively similar in functioning.

6.2.9.1   Gross-Motor

This scale is related to, but is more focused than, the Physical scale of Developmental Profile II (Section 6.2.2.3). There are 42 items of the following type: sits, creeps, crawls, walks, runs, jumps, uses stairs, climbs, hops, throws, catches, rides bicycle/tricycle (raw score range 0 to 84).

6.2.9.2   Interpersonal

This scale is related to, but is more focused than, the Social scale of Developmental Profile II (Section 6.2.2.4). There are 17 items of the following type: wants to please others, labels own emotions, imitates gestures and tasks, names familiar people, knows family relationships, laughs/smiles appropriately, responds to others' good fortune, initiates topic of interest to others, responds to hints, gets gifts for others, remembers anniversaries, has preference for some friends, has best friend, has regular group of friends (raw score range 0 to 34).

6.2.9.3 Play

This scale is concerned with how the child uses play and leisure time for solitary activities and requiring interaction with others. There are 18 items of the following type: plays with toys, uses household objects for play, shows interest in other's activities, plays interaction game, plays group game, takes part in make-believe activities, plays board games, follows rules for games, shares, has preferences for TV programmes, uses radio/TV for information and news, has hobbies, plays non-school sports, attends evening school and non-school events (raw score range 0 to 36).

6.2.9.4 Activities of Daily Living

Similar to the Self-Help scale of Developmental Profile II (Section 6.2.2.5), this scale is concerned with independence in activities of daily living. There are 36 items of the following type: sucks/chews, eats solid food, drinks from cup/glass, sucks through straw, gets water from tap, uses spoon/fork/knife, indicates soiled pants, urinates/defecates in potty/WC, toilet trained, cares for toilet needs, bathes self, washes/dries face, dries body, bathes/showers/dries, cleans teeth, cares for nose, cares for hair, cares for fingernails, covers mouth while sneezing, avoids contagious people, looks after own health, removes clothing, puts on footwear, ties laces, puts on clothes, dresses completely, uses fasteners and zippers, changes clothes, chooses clothes (raw score range 0 to 72).

6.2.9.5 Attention and Control

For each of eight items describing a particular situation, the child is scored on a five point scale depending on the length of attention span and the extent of self control. The eight items are as follows; listening in a group, engaged in an easy task with supervision, engaged in a difficult task without supervision, concentrating when distractions are present, quietening down after active period, taking turns, distruptive behaviour in a group, temper control (raw score range 8 to 40).

6.2.10 Behaviour Problems

A questionnaire was posted to the mother of each child. One section of the questionnaire is a 13 item check-list of problem behaviours: thumb/finger sucking, bed wetting, eating problems, sleeping problems, nail biting, tics/twitches, crying, teeth grinding, concentration problems, temper tantrums, withdrawal, rocking, self-injurious behaviour. The child is scored 0, 1, or 2 on each item by the mother depending on whether the child often, sometimes or never demonstrates the problem behaviour. The sum of scores gives an overall index of the extent of the behaviour problems (raw score range 0 to 26 indicating no behaviour problems).

6.3 SELECTION OF THE BIRMINGHAM GROUP AND THE TIMING OF THE ASSESSMENTS

The requirements of conductive education dictate the make-up of a participating group (Section 3, Section 4). Not all children with cerebral palsy can participate and benefit from conductive education, hence children must be screened before they can be accepted. Those who are suitable must then be allocated to specifically composed groups because the make-up of the group is important for the practice of conductive education.

The establishment of conductive education at the Birmingham Institute was under the close supervision of the Pető Institute which desired full control over the selection of children. The research project had no role in the selection and the Institutes were not fettered by possible research requirements. The selection proceeded in three stages.

6.3.1 Stage 1

In the first stage, children were put forward for possible invitation to Stage 2 by agencies and parents in response to a widely circulated 'Notice of Admission'. The wording of the notice was the responsibility of the Birmingham Foundation for Conductive Education which made use of information and instructions from the Pető Institute. The notice included the following criteria:

i.   having a form of cerebral palsy.

ii.   birthdates between 1 January 1983 and 31 August 1985.

iii. not also suffering from profound mental handicap, blindness, autism, continuous ill health, continuous fits or medication that could seriously affect ability to participate in the programme.

iv.   already living within daily travelling distance of the Birmingham Institute.

Criterion iv was imposed because the Birmingham Institute is non-residential and the maximum travelling time was set at 45 minutes. The catchment area therefore covered the whole of the West Midlands Metropolitan County, as well as the proximate areas of the neighbouring county councils of Hereford and Worcester, Staffordshire, and Warwickshire.

According to the Birmingham Institute, only criteria i, ii and iv were firmly adhered to in Stage 1. For example, if a child had spina bifida, was too old or too young, or lived too far away, an invitation to attend Stage 2 was not given.

It is recognised that many of the terms in criterion iii are imprecise, but they are the terms which were used in the 'Notice of Admission' and are therefore repeated here. Factors in criterion iii anticipate assessments carried out in Stage 2 and the Birmingham Institute provided an invitation to attend even if there were doubts about suitability.

Neither the language spoken in the child's home, the severity of physical disability, previous educational experiences, nor previous medical or surgical treatment, were factors determining initial eligibility.

6.3.2   Stage 2

Only conductors could judge whether a child is suitable for conductive education. Accordingly, in the second stage, pairs of senior conductors travelled from Budapest to carry out their own assessments of the children put forward in Stage 1. Information from three sources was used in the assessment.

i.   Medical records were consulted for information relating to diagnosis, history of epilepsy, medication and surgery.

ii.   A questionnaire was filled out by parents providing information on the mother's pregnancy, the child at birth, and the child's early motor development.

iii.   Direct observation and assessment of the child without the use of physical aids or appliances took place. A number of aspects were included depending on the nature of the child, and the following is a summary of headings; a. general description of the child, b. assessment of lying down, c. four-point kneeling, d. high kneeling, e. standing, f. reflexes, g. sitting, h. use of pen and paper. While the assessments were carried out, the conductors subjectively evaluated each child's general mental ability, and the ability to make contact, and communicate, with the conductors and the parents. The assessment of the ability to 'make contact', is considered an important part of the evaluation. The parent was also asked about any previous surgery on the child.

On the basis of information gained from the above sources, and against a background of following many children in conductive education, the conductors decided which of the children put forward were suitable for conductive education.

The conductors also provided a diagnosis of each child's condition because they did not necessarily agree with diagnoses in the medical records, and a 'severity rating' (severe, moderate, mild) for children found suitable for conductive education. This rating, devised by the conductors, is a judgement mainly concerning the severity of the physical disability but also a prognosis about the ease with which the disability could be overcome with conductive education. Such ratings are carried out at the Pető Institute but not routinely. They are often not recorded because of a desire not to 'label' children especially in the early years.

6.3.3 Stage 3

Not all children found suitable for conductive education in Stage 2 could be accepted at the Birmingham Institute because of the limited number of places. There was provision for only one group and the fact that the make-up of a group is important for the practice of conductive education necessitated a third stage in which the conductors were again involved. They applied their own criteria and judgement in the final decision about who would be enrolled and took into account the mixture of children already enrolled when making decisions about subsequent intakes. The basis for their decisions is largely unknown except that the inclusion of a range of abilities and personalities is said to be crucial.

6.3.4 Intakes

The 20 children who originally took part in the research project were enrolled in three intakes. Ten children in Intake 1 began their conductive education at the Pető Institute in Budapest in January 1988 and remained there for five months. Eight children in Intake 2 were enrolled in Birmingham in September and October 1988 where they joined Intake 1 which had by that time returned from Budapest. There were two children in Intake 3 enrolled in September 1989 and January 1990 respectively.

The 20 children were assessed annually for the research project during a period close to the nominal date of 1 January and they were treated as a single group even though they were enrolled in three intakes at different times. The rationale for this treatment needs to be explained.

The first full research assessment of Intake 1 (n=10) and Intake 2 (n=8) took place over a period close to 1 January 1989 at which time Intake 1 had received 5 months more conductive education than Intake 2 (January 1989-May 1989 inclusive). There is evidence, however, that Intake 1 had not benefited from this extra conductive education making it valid to combine data from the two intakes. This evidence will now be reviewed.

The conductors provided a 'severity rating' (severe, moderate, mild) of the children at the time of their enrolment (Section 6.3.2). If these ratings are converted to 1, 2, and 3 respectively, the two intakes did not differ in their severity at the time of their enrolment (Mann Whitney U Test, $U=25$, $N_1=8$, $n_2=10$, ns).

By January 1 1989 when the children were being assessed for the research project the two intakes were of similar chronological age (Table 6.1). Parents were questioned to establish the date on which the children were first exposed to some form of intervention of an educational kind and to establish the subsequent history of educational experiences. The period since first becoming involved in education was calculated and it was established that the two intakes had been exposed to educational experiences for a similar period of time (Table 6.1), albeit Intake 1 had, of course, received more conductive education than Intake 2.

The two intakes can be compared on a subset of the full battery of assessments which was used subsequently to identify a matched group in Manchester: age-differential on the Self-Help, Social and Communication scales of Developmental Profile II according to parent report; independence in 18 activities of a Gross-Motor Assessment according to parent estimate; preferred-hand and nonpreferred-hand function on a direct test. The two intakes did not differ on any of the assessments (Table 6.1).

Reviewing the above, Intake 1 and Intake 2 received a similar severity rating by the conductors when they were enrolled and therefore commenced their conductive education with overall similar motor disabilities. At the time of their assessment for the research, the two intakes were of similar chronological age and had previously experienced some form of education for a similar period of time, but Intake 1 had received 5 months more conductive education than Intake 2. The two intakes, however, had similar abilities in a range of domains. On the evidence available, however, Intake 1 had not benefited more as a result of its extra conductive education that Intake 2 had from other education over an equivalent period. No distinction will, therefore, be made between the data from Intakes 1 and 2.

The first full research assessment of Intake 3 ($n=2$) took place in a period centred on 1 January 1990 close to when the children were enrolled which was approximately a year after Intake 2. Children in Intake 3 are approximately a year younger than those in the first two intakes and their data will be pooled with the data of Intakes 1 and 2 gathered a year earlier.

6.3.5 Timing of Assessments for the Birmingham Group

The timing of assessments of children in the Birmingham Institute is summarised as follows, the nominal date being within the period during which assessments were carried out:

Time 1 Assessment   Intakes 1 and 2   1 January 1989
                                    Intake 3   1 January 1990

Time 2 Assessment	Intakes 1 and 2	1 January 1990
	Intake 3	1 January 1991
Time 3 Assessment	Intakes 1 and 2	1 January 1991
	Intake 3	1 January 1992

In practice, the chronological age of the children at every assessment was recorded to confirm that assessments were separated by a 12 month period, and also to confirm that the Birmingham and Manchester groups were of similar age at Time 1, Time 2 and Time 3 assessments.

6.4 SELECTION OF A MATCHED GROUP OF CHILDREN RECEIVING ALTERNATIVE BRITISH PROGRAMMES OF SPECIAL EDUCATION IN GREATER MANCHESTER AND THE TIMING OF THE ASSESSMENTS

There were severe problems for the research team from the start in identifying a comparison group of children enrolled in alternative programmes of British special education. First, as outlined in Section 6.3 the Pető Institute working with the Birmingham Foundation was responsible for screening and selecting children for the Birmingham Institute. The research team had no control over the selection, and the three stage process depended on staff from the Pető Institute using unpublished and nonstandardised procedures and criteria. Second the timetable for establishing the Birmingham Institute and the timetable for designing and implementing the evaluation were not coordinated. The first instake of 10 children was enrolled long before the research methodologies were established and the second intake of 8 children was enrolled scarcely before the assessment package was established and before a methodology for selecting comparison children had been designed. Third, it took time to establish successful working relationships with those concerned with providing conductive education; namely, the Pető Institute, Birmingham Foundation and Birmingham Institute. Against this background, the procedure employed during 1989 which lead to the eventual identification of a comparison group will be described.

Two factors initially determined where the search for a comparison group would be focussed. First, as outlined in Section 6.3, the Birmingham Institute had already enrolled children from a wide catchment area using a non-random procedure. The residual pool of children within the catchment area might be biased, hence it was desirable to select comparison children from outside the area. Second, the Department of Education and Science (the sponsor of the research) supplied the names of local authorities which, it was believed, provided good services for cerebral palsied children and it was desirable to have comparison children enrolled in well regarded programes of education.

The process which eventually lead to the identification of a comparison group in November 1989 began in June 1988 when letters were sent to pairs of education and health authorities suggested by the Department of Education and Science (Appendix 6.1). [It will be noted that this letter makes reference to an experimental design which was subsequently not implemented.] There were also other authorities and individual schools interested in providing comparison groups and some of these made initial contact with the research team. There was a period of negotiation with many of these authorities and schools extending over nearly 12 months, during which time details of the experimental design and methodologies were established.

By May 1989 three key features of the research had been established. First, the evaluation would involve the identification of groups of children initially matched as closely as possible to the 18 children then enrolled in the Birmingham Institute, but receiving alternative special education. Second, the development of the matched group of children would be documented as broadly as possible using general assessments of function not specifically related to the objectives of the different programmes of education (Section 6.2). Third, the comparison group would be fully assessed for the first time approximately one year later than the first assessment of the Birmingham children and therefore had to be a year younger than the Birmingham children.

The procedure for identifying children matched to those in the Birmingham Institute needed to be as similar as possible to the procedure used at the Institute. Children had been put forward for possible screening in response to a 'Notice of Admission' which included particular criteria (Stage 1, Section 6.3.1). Those that seemed to satisfy the written criteria were then screened by the Pető Institute for suitabllility for conductive education using unpublished and nonstandardized procedures (Stage 2, Section 6.3.2). The Pető Institute also decided which children would be enrolled so that a cohort would be established suitable for the practice of conductive education (Stage 3, Section 6.3.3). Clearly, comparison children would have to be 'suitable for conductive education' (albeit receiving alternative education), the Pető Institute would therefore have to be involved in the selection of comparison children and there would have to be controls to ensure that the selection was unprejudiced (Section 6.4.2). Negotiations with the Pető Institute began in March 1989.

6.4.1   Stage 1

Cooperating authorities were provided with initial criteria similar to those in the Birmingham Institute's 'Notice of Admission' (Section 6.3.1).

i.   Having a form of cerebral palsy.

ii.   Birthdates between 1 January 1984 and 31 August 1986, one year later than the Birmingham group because the first assessment of the comparison children would take place one year later than the first assessment of the Birmingham group.

iii. Not also suffering from profound mental handicap, blindness, autism, continuous ill health, continuous fits or medication that could seriously affect ability to participate in a programme of education.

The authorities consulted their registers and records for children who might satisfy these criteria. Factors in criterion iii anticipate assessments carried out in Stage 2 and the authorities were encouraged to include as many children as possible even if there was doubt about suitability. Letters were sent to parents seeking their consent to the study. (Appendix 6.2. It will be noted that children were originally to be followed for three years rather than two years).

6.4.2   Stage 2

Senior conductors from the Pető Institute in Budapest carried out their own assessments of the children using three sources of information described in Section 6.3.2. One of the conductors had been engaged in the selection of the first intake in Birmingham, which helped to provide consistency in the methods and criteria employed.

To reduce the risk of bias in selection, conductors' assessments were carried out 'blind' using an agreed procedure. Children were brought from other areas in England for assessment, not as potential comparisons, but for acceptance into the Pető Institute in Budapest. These children were included among the potential comparison children. The plan was that the conductors would not know at the time of their assessment the full name of the child, and whether they were assessing for conductive education in Budapest or for inclusion in the comparison group.

If medical information was required which could have revealed the identity of the child, it was supplied by a medical officer and the identity of the child concealed. In the case of potential comparison children, the Local Health Authority had given informed consent to the study being carried out in its area, and doctors responsible for the children provided any information required, after parents had individually consented to information being provided. In the case of the children being assessed for the Pető Institute many attended the assessment with medical notes and a doctor was usually available to supplement the notes with an additional history and examination if necessary. Among children who eventually made up the comparison group, their identities and the true purpose of the assessment was concealed from the conductors in all but two cases until the conductors had provided the following information: their judgement of suitability for conductive education, their diagnosis of a child's condition, a 'severity rating' described in Section 6.3.2 and, where appropriate, reasons for judging a child unsuitable for conductive education.

The research team carried out separate assessments on all children put forward for Stage 2. These assessments were a subset of the full battery (Section 6.2) and were the same as those used for comparing Intake 1 and Intake 2 of the Birmingham group at Time 1: age-differential on the Self-Help, Social and Communication scales of Developmental Profile II according to parent report; independence in 18 activities of a Gross-Motor assessment according to parent estimate; preferred-hand and nonpreferred-hand function on a direct test.

Stage 2 assessments were generally carried out in the special schools in which the potential comparison children were enrolled. Each child was generally accompanied by one or both parents.

6.4.2.1   Stage 2 Procedure for Potential Comparison Children

The procedure for potential comparison children had the following general form. The child and parent attended a short initial interview with one of the research team, which was introduced with background of the following general form: ' . . . the Department of Education and Science has commissioned the University of Birmingham to follow the group of children enrolled in the Birmingham Institute for Conductive Education. The purpose is to see how the children develop in this new programme of education, and this work has already begun. The Department is also interested in the University following groups of children away from Birmingham in other programmes of education to see how they develop. The research team has been advised to come to this particular school because the Department has a high regard for the programmes being offered, and the children might make progress comparable to that of the children receiving conductive education. The question is whether conductive education has anything to offer over and above what is already being achieved in existing programmes of education. The first task of the research team is to identify children who are like the Birmingham children. The school has put forward children who may be similar to the Birmingham children as far as they know, and the research team has come to see for itself, and to carry out a short assessment. The other people who are involved are conductors from the Pető Institute one of whom chose the Birmingham children. They have been invited to see the children, and to inform us whether, in their opinion, the children are like those who were chosen for Birmingham'.

The order of the assessment was then described. First, the parent and child went to see the conductors who assessed the child and talked to the parent. Second, a member of the research team interviewed the parent in relation to the three scales of the Development Profile II. Third, the parent and child came back to the first member of the research team who interviewed the parent in relation to the child's gross-motor independence, and carried out the test of hand function. The parent was asked if there were any questions about the assessments. It was then explained that after all the assessments were completed, decisions would be made about whether children had been found who were like those in the Birmingham group. If so the parent would be approached again for consent to allow us to follow the child's progress. It was emphasised that no attempt would be made by the research team to change the programme of education already being offered. This would involve a certain commitment from the parent, and more information would be provided about what the future assessments would entail.

6.4.2.2 Stage 2 Procedure for Children Assessed for Acceptance into the Pető Institute

The procedure for children being assessed for the acceptance to the Pető Institute was slightly different. The child and parent attended a short initial interview with one of the research team which was introduced with background of the following general form: ' . . . the main purpose is to meet with the Hungarian conductors who will carry out their assessment but there are also other people we would like you to meet. The Department of Education and Science has commissioned the University of Birmingham to follow the progress of children at the Birmingham Institute for Conductive Education. The department is interested in knowing what type of child is suitable for conductive education, and the type of child that is rejected. Hence, the research team would like to assess the children seen by the conductors to gain information to help in the research effort'. The agreement of the parent was obtained to carry out interviews as well as a short assessment of the child (the same as that carried out for potential comparison children).

The order of the assessments was then described. First, the parent and child would see the conductors. They would carry out their assessment but would then need time to decide on whether the child was suitable for conductive education. The parent should not at this stage question the conductors.

This was the method adopted to prevent the parent revealing to the conductors the identity of the child and the true purpose of the assessment. Second, immediately following the assessment the parent was interviewed by a member of the research team in relation to the three scales of the Developmental Profile II. Third, the parent and child came back to the first member of the research team for the interview regarding the child's gross-motor independence and also for the test of hand function. It was explained that the conductors would then be able to see the parent again, and a second meeting would be arranged at which time the conductors would tell the parent whether conductive education was appropriate for the child, and possibly when a place would become available at the Pető Institute. Generally, a member of the research team would first go to the conductors and tell them that a particular parent and child was returning (this, of course, was after the conductors had already provided the information for the research). The conductors did not know that the particular child was one being assessed for possible acceptance to the Pető Institute, indicating that procedures for the 'blind' assessment were successful.

6.4.3 Stage 3

Only children judged suitable for conductive education were further considered for inclusion in a comparison group. The aim in stage 3 was to identify a sufficiently large cohort of 'suitable' children (not less than 10 children and hopefully as many as 20 children) matched to the 18 children then in the Birmingham Institute on the conductors' opinion on diagnosis, the conductors' severity rating and the research team's assessments.

Screening assessments were first carried out in Bradford and Liverpool in July 1989. Only eight and ten children respecively passed stage 2, and neither cohort was well matched to the Birmingham group.

Supplementary assessments were carried out in Bradford and a new round of assessments in Trafford in September 1989. There were now eleven children passing stage 2 in Bradford, and nine children in Trafford but neither cohort was well matched to the Birmingham group.

It became apparent that the Birmingham Institute had been so selective in its choice of children and sampling had taken place from such a wide catchment area that no similar comparison group could be found in any single authority or school. It was clear that a comparison group would have to be drawn from a catchment area similar in size to that of the Birmingham Institute and encompassing more than one authority and school.

Using groups already identified in Trafford and Liverpool as foci, an attempt was made to form a Greater Manchester and a Merseyside group (respectively) by carrying out a further round of screening assessments in neighbouring authorities in November 1989. There was now a total of 26 children passing in Stage 2 in Greater Manchester (Trafford, Oldham and Wigan authorities) and 16 children in Merseyside (Liverpool, Knowsley and Wirral authorities).

Because of resource limitations, it was subsequently decided to follow only one comparison group, namely from Greater Manchester, and the procedure by which 20 children were selected from the 26 passing Stage 2 will now be described.

One main variable was chosen to match comparison children to the Birmingham group, namely the Self-Help scale of Developmental Profile

II (Section 6.2.2.5). This scale has items concerned with feeding, dressing, toileting and household chores, and a child passes or fails on an item depending on whether the parent says the child can or cannot exhibit the behaviour described. While the scale is specifically concerned with the child's independence in activities of daily living, such independence is likely to be related to physical ability, self-motivation and social development. Initial assessments of all three intakes in Birmingham (N=19, one parent was unavailable for interview) show that developmental age on the Self-Help scale correlates with the following; developmental age on the Social scale (Section 6.2.2.4, $r_s = + 0.70$), parent report of gross-motor independence (Section 6.2.7, $r_s = + 0.61$), direct assessment of the preferred-hand (Section 6.2.6.3, $r_s = + 0.70$), conductor's severity rating (Section 6.3.2, $r_s = + 0.58$). Selecting children on the basis of scores on the Self-Help scale, therefore, also takes some account of other aspects of functioning which are not only correlated to independence in activities of daily living but also would be considered important in any programme of education for physically disabled children.

The 18 children in Birmingham to which the comparison group were to be matched ranged from –1 to –60 months age differential on the Self-Help scale.

The 26 Greater Manchester children ranged from +34 to –61 months age-differential. Three children with positive age differentials were excluded, and three children with a diagnosis of hemiplegia were also excluded because there were no children with this diagnosis in the Birmingham group. There now remained 20 children; 10 enrolled in one school, and 5 each enrolled in two other schools.

The 20 Greater Manchester children (to be referred to as the Manchester group) can now be compared to the 18 Birmingham children on the range of variables used in the screening process. The first full assessment of the Birmingham group took place over a period near to the nominal date of 1 January 1989, while the first full assessment of the Manchester group would take place near to the nominal date of 1 January 1990. At these set dates the Manchester group is younger than the Birmingham group (Table 6.2) indicating that future annual assessments in Manchester should take place after assessments in Birmingham to ensure that at Time 1, Time 2 and Time 3 Assessments, the two groups are of similar chronological age. The conductors provided diagnoses of the children in one of four categories (quadriplegic, diplegic, athetoid, ataxic) and the two groups are not dissimilar in the frequency of those categories (Table 6.2). There is no significant difference between groups in the frequency of the conductor's severity ratings (severe, moderate, mild, Table 6.2). The apparent difference in frequency may be the result of inaccuracy in the conductor's rating (Section 6.6.3), a conclusion supported by later findings of group equivalence on a broad range of measures of fine-motor and gross-motor functioning (Section 6.8). according to parent report on Developmental Profile II, children in the Manchester group have significantly lower age differentials than the Birmingham group on the Social scale but the two groups do not differ significantly on the Self-Help or Communication scale (Table 6.2). Finally, the two groups do not differ significantly on parent report of gross-motor independence or on the direct assessment of preferred-hand and nonpreferred-hand function (Table 6.2).

The above data ranging over a number of conductor assessments and research assessments, and over direct and indirect measure of functional abilities in different domains, are strong support for the conclusion that the Birmingham and Manchester groups were matched on most of the criteria chosen for matching. This is not meant to imply that the groups were identical, or that they would not differ on other variables, but given the high level of variability among children within the diagnostic category of 'cerebral palsy', this initial indication of group matching was as good as could be hoped for.

6.4.4 Timing of Assessments for the Manchester Group

The timing of the assessments of children in the Manchester group is as follows, the nominal data being within the period during which assessments were carried out:

Time 1 assessment   1 January 1990
Time 2 assessment   1 January 1991
Time 3 assessment   1 January 1992

In practice, the chronological age of the children at every assessment was recorded to confirm that assessments were separated by a 12 month period, and also to confirm that the Birmingham and Manchester groups were of similar age at Time 1, Time 2 and Time 3 assessments.

6.5 FINAL CONSTITUTION OF THE BIRMINGHAM AND MANCHESTER GROUPS

Early in the evaluation, one child in the Birmingham group who was part of the cohort for which comparisons were being sought in Manchester, was withdrawn from the Birmingham Institute by the parents for reasons other than being dissatisfied with conductive education. The conductors, on the other hand, were not unwilling to let the child be withdrawn because little progress was being made, the onset of epilepsy was suspected, and there was a growing doubt about the suitability of the child for conductive education.

It was anticipated that children might leave the Institute for a variety of reasons during the period of the research evaluation. The plan was to continue documenting the development of the children because they would have already received a significant amount of conductive education (certainly more than the comparison children) and one might expect a carry-over of any benefits during subsequent years in alternative education.

Unfortunately for the evaluation project, the parents not only withdrew the child from the Institute, but also expressed a wish to be no longer be associated with the research. Difficulties for the evaluation were compounded by the fact that the child was very different from any other child enrolled at the Institute and considerable effort had been expended on finding similar children for the comparison group. On many of the assessments there was no other child in the Institute performing any where near as poorly and it is difficult to find any assessment on which another child received an equal or lower score.

The wide ranging nature of the child's severe difficulties can be illustrated with Time 1 assessment data (Table 6.3). Taking parent report on all five scales of Developmental Profile II and calculating mean age-differentials it can be seen that the child not only functioned poorly according to the parent but also functioned well below the next eight children rank ordered on mean age-differential. The small standard deviation for Child 14 shows that this child had difficulties relevant to all scales, while the large standard deviations for the other children indicate that they only had difficulties in relation to some scales. A further illustration comes from the full range of Time 1 direct assessments covering cognition, speech, fine-motor and gross-motor functioning. The individual direct tests yield 15 direct measures of functioning. Child 14 was unique in scoring above zero on only five of these direct measures; the child seemed motivated but was incapable of performing.

Even though Child 14 was clearly very different from any other child in the Institute, the child would have remained one of the Birmingham group if the parents had not withdrawn the child from the evaluation. This withdrawal together with experiences gathered in the Time 1 assessments in Manchester, prompted a revision of the make-up of the Manchester group.

As the Manchester group was being assessed at Time 1 there seemed to be three children who were like Birmingham Child 14 discussed above. All three were scoring uniformly poorly on indirect assessments and seemed motivated but incapable of a measurable response on most of the direct tests. Illustrative data are given in Table 6.4 which gives the mean age-differential on five scales of Developmental Profile II (parent report) and the number of above zero scores on 15 direct measures of functioning for the three children (Child 31, 38, 43). Corresponding data from the next six children rank ordered on mean age-differential is also given (Child 41, 34, 39, 49, 37, 40).

It will be noted that Child 41 and Child 49 gave a mixed picture. The former scored very poorly on Developmental Profile II but produced measurable responses on the majority of direct tests. The latter did not score very poorly on Developmental Profile II but failed to score above zero on the direct tests not because the child was incapable but rather because it was impossible to gain the child's attention and cooperation.

In the interest of establishing a closer initial match between the Manchester and Birmingham groups, three Manchester children (Child 31, 38, 43) were excluded from the comparison because they were like Child 14 on dual criteria; ie, globally low scores on indirect assessments of function and global inability to produce measurable responses on direct tests. Accordingly, data from 19 children in Birmingham and 17 children in Manchester are included in the main analyses.

The progress of all children enrolled in the Birmingham Institute is compared to the progress of a small subset of children enrolled in schools in Greater Manchester. This provides a test of the effectiveness of conductive education against a standard provided by a matched group of children in United Kingdom special education. The comparison does not provide a general test of the effectiveness of United Kingdom special education because only a small subset of children in the schools is studied. Hence, conclusions on the effectiveness of United Kingdom special education can only be relevant to children who would be accepted for conductive education and are not relevant to the larger number of children enrolled in the Manchester schools.

6.6 PSYCHOMETRICS, PRINCIPAL-COMPONENTS ANALYSIS, DATA REDUCTION

6.6.1 Introduction

Parts of the assessment battery discussed in Section 6.2 make use of previously published tests, some of which report reliability and validity data. Other parts of the battery were designed for the present evaluation and there was only limited opportunity to carry out desirable psychometric investigations. One aim of the present section is to direct the reader to previously published psychometric data and also to report the limited amount of new data that was collected.

The second aim is to report on intercorrelations in Time 1 criterion-referenced data. Such data show whether chronological age is related to function in cerebral palsy and also give support to the validity of the assessments as tests in cerebral palsy. There are also data concerning the validity of the conductor's 'severity rating' of the children (Section 6.3.2).

The intercorrelation data reveal relationships between diverse parts of the assessment battery. A Principal-Components Analysis was carried out on

Time 1 criterion-referenced data to summarise the pattern of interrelationship among the variables. The third aim is to report the results of this analysis, along with the method used for combining subsets of variables in the calculation of global measures of functioning.

6.6.2   Psychometrics

Developmental Profile II, Pictorial Test of Intelligence, Reynell Developmental Language Scales and Vineland Adaptive Behaviour Scales have been published with manuals which report acceptable data on reliability (eg., test-retest reliability, inter-rater reliability) and concurrent validity. The Frenchay Dysarthria Assessment, Fletcher Time-by-Count Test of Diadochokinetic Syllable Rate, Preverbal Communication Schedule and Edinburgh Articulation Test have also been published but with limited or no data on reliability and validity.

The other parts of the assessment battery including the Achievement Test, Fine-Motor Assessment, Gross-Motor Assessment, Attention and Control and Behaviour Problems were modifications of previously published tests or were newly developed for the current project. There was insufficient time to establish fully the psychometric properties of these tests, none of them have been published elsewhere even in their present form, and this report is the only source of information about them. The purpose here is to discuss the limited amount of psychometric data that was obtained.

The first and second intakes of the Birmingham Group were retested on part of the assessment battery in June 1989 which was in the period between Time 1 and Time 2 assessments. Parents were interviewed in relation to Developmental Profile II, the children were directly assessed on the Fine Motor Assessment and conductors were interviewed in relation to the Adaptive Behaviour scales. While the period between the Time 1 and this interim assessment was around five months and is, therefore, rather long for an investigation of test-retest reliability, the two sets of data give at least a preliminary and conservative indication of reliability of these tests when applied to children with cerebral palsy. One child from Intake 2 was lost from the study while one parent failed to attend the interview for Developmental Profile II at Time 1, hence, the data are from 17 or 16 children depending on the test. Despite the small number of children, the long period between assessments, and statistically significant changes in mean performance of the group, the correlation coefficients for Developmental Profile II (Table 6.5) and the Adaptive Behaviour scales (Table 6.7) ranging from 0.54 to 0.92, support the reliability data published in the test manuals. On the other hand, the Fine-Motor Assessment which has not been previously published, yielded correlation coefficients (Table 6.6) ranging from 0.54 to 0.94, giving a preliminary indication that this assessment yields reliable data from children with cerebral palsy.

The Fine-Motor Assessment was video-recorded with a 0.1 sec time base and criterion-referenced scores were taken from the recordings according to written criteria. Two judges independently derived data from the recordings of the Time 1 assessments of Intakes 1 and 2 of the Birmingham Group. The correlation coefficients given in Table 6.8 show that inter-rater reliability is very high.

Similarly, the Gross-Motor assessment was video-recorded with a 0.1 sec time base and criterion-referenced scores were taken from the recordings according to written criteria. Two judges independently derived the data from the recordings of the Time 1 assessments of five children in the Manchester Group and the data in Table 6.9 show high inter-rater reliability.

An investigation was carried out into the incidence of 'floor' and 'ceiling' effects in criterion-referenced data gathered at Time 1 and Time 3, ie., a tally was made of the number of children who functioned so poorly that they were given the lowest possible score, and the number of children who functioned so well that they were given the highest possible score. The five physical variables—Hip Mobility, Hamstring Extensibility, Height, Weight, Neurological assessment—were not considered because it was only meaningful to include functional variables. In addition, the four Pre-Verbal Communication variables—Motor Control 3, Receptive Non-Verbal, Expressive Non-Verbal, Receptive Verbal—were not considered because these had been included in the test battery primarily to document the progress of the relatively few non-verbal children and it was anticipated that the majority of children who would be expressing themselves verbally would be functioning at the ceiling of these tests. This leaves 38 criterion-referenced functional variables on which the 35 children were assessed at Time 1 and Time 3. The incidence of floor and ceiling effects at Time 1 was five per cent and one per cent respectively, while the incidence of floor and ceiling effects at Time 3 was four per cent and three per cent respectively. It is concluded, therefore, that the data set is effectively free of floor effects and is also effectively free of ceiling effects except for the Pre-Verbal Communication variables.

6.6.3   Intercorrelations in Time 1 Data

There was a fairly wide range in chronological age among the 35 children in the Birmingham and Manchester groups, eg., chronological age at the Time 1 Fine-Motor assessment ranged from 44 to 71 months. Chronological age was not, however, a covariate of raw test data because performance correlated poorly with chronological age in these children with cerebral palsy. The full set of correlations relating chronological age to functional criterion-referenced raw scores at Time 1 is given in Appendix 6.3.

An investigation of the relationship between chronological age at Time 1 and change over the Time 1 to Time 3 period on the same set of functional criterion-referenced raw scores, yielded infrequent (a total of seven) and scattered correlations which were statistically significant albeit low (range $r = 0.35$ to $r = 0.50$). Some correlations were positive indicating that older children tended to make better progress than younger children, while other correlations were negative indicating that older children tended to make worse progress than younger children. Giving the infrequency of the significant correlations and their low magnitude, it was concluded that chronological age would not be considered to be a covariate of change in function.

The many variables yielded by the assessment battery covered the following domains of function; general cognition, receptive and expressive language, fine-motor functioning, gross-motor functioning, social behaviour, activities of daily living. It is useful to examine the relationship between variables within a domain for evidence of concurrent validity of the individual tests. For example, a range of direct and indirect tests were used to assess gross-motor functioning and if the set of variables obtained at Time 1 correlated, it would be possible to conclude that the tests were valid measures of gross-motor functioning in cerebral palsy.

General Cognition. The Academic scale of Developmental Profile II yields an indirect measure of general cognitive ability according to parent report of the childrens' functioning, while the Pictorial Test of Intelligence yields a direct measure of general cognitive ability. The correlation between raw scores from the two tests at Time 1 was 0.50 which is broadly in line with concurrent validity data reported in the manuals relevant to these two tests.

Receptive and Expressive Language. There are 10 tests in the battery which directly and indirectly assess five aspects of receptive and expressive language; receptive non-verbal communication, expressive non-verbal communication, motor control of the speech apparatus, receptive verbal communication, expressive verbal communication. The Communication scale of Developmental Profile II yields an indirect measure according to parent report which encompasses most of the above aspects of language. The other nine tests yield more specific measures. The Receptive Non-Verbal scale and the Expressive Non-Verbal scale involve mainly an indirect assessment according to parent report of the abilities to understand non-verbal communication and to communicate non-verbally. There are four assessments of ability to control the speech apparatus, some direct and some indirect; Motor Control 1, Motor Control 2, Motor Control 3 and Articulation. There are two assessments of receptive verbal communication; the Pictorial Test of Intelligence which gives a direct assessment of general cognitive ability also requires good verbal understanding, while the Receptive Verbal scale is an indirect assessment of verbal understanding.

Finally, the Expressive Verbal scale directly assesses expressive verbal communication. The correlation matrix based on Time 1 raw score data, given in Table 6.10, show a pattern of intercorrelations which give evidence for concurrent validity of these tests. The Communication scale of Developmental Profile II, the global measure of receptive and expressive language, correlates with all nine specific measures. Receptive Non-Verbal, Pictorial Test of Intelligence and Receptive Verbal correlate with one another indicating, perhaps, a general receptive language ability among these children. The four measures of ability to control the speech apparatus correlate with one another and also with the Expressive Verbal scale, as one might expect.

Fine-Motor.   Eight tests are concerned with fine-motor functioning. The Physical scale of Developmental Profile II gives an indirect measure according to parent report and it also covers gross-motor abilities. The other seven tests yield direct measures of fine-motor functioning; Fine-Motor Independence, Object Transfer 1, Object Transfer 2, Manipulation, Two-Hand Coordination, Placement and Drawing. The correlation matrix based on Time 1 raw score data, given in Table 6.11, includes many statistically significant correlations which is evidence for concurrent validity of these tests. The two paper-and-pencil tasks correlate highly with one another but not particularly well with other fine-motor tasks indicating, perhaps, that they require different kinds of abilities.

Gross-Motor.   Eleven tests are concerned with gross-motor functioning. The Physical scale of Developmental Profile II and the Gross-Motor scale of Adaptive Behaviour give indirect measures according to parent and teacher report respectively. The other nine tests yield direct measures of gross-motor functioning; Postural Independence, Position Changing Independence, Crawling Independence, Walking Independence, Preferred Locomotion Independence, Position Changing, Crawling, Walking and Preferred Locomotion. Table 6.12 gives the correlation matix based on Time 1 raw score data. The many high correlations are evidence for concurrent validity of these tests, the exception being Preferred Locomotion Independence which does not correlate highly with the other tests.

Correlations between conductors' severity rating and parent report on the Physical scale of Developmental Profile II, and between severity rating and teacher report on the Gross-Motor scale of Adaptive Behaviour, are $r_s = 0.71$ and $r_s = 0.74$ respectively. Clearly, there is broad agreement between the conductor's assessment of the children and the two research assessments of the children, although there is disagreement on individual children; eg., children rated 'severe' by the conductors who function better according to the two research scales than children rated 'moderate' by the conductors'. It seems that the conductors' severity rating is an inaccurate indicator of function. The apparent, albeit non-significant, difference between the Birmingham and Manchester groups in the numbers of children judged 'severe', moderate' and 'mild' (Table 6.2) may be the result of inaccuracy in the rating, a conclusion supported by later research data showing group equivalence (Section 6.8).

Social. The Social scale of Developmental Profile II yields an indirect measure according to parent report while the Interpersonal scale and Play scale of Adaptive Behaviour give indirect measures according to teacher report. Data in Table 6.13 show that the three tests correlate well.

Activities of Daily Living. The Self-Help scale of Developmental Profile II and the Activities of Daily Living scale of Adaptive Behaviour give indirect measures according to parent and teacher report, respectively, which correlate ($r = 0.75$).

6.6.4   Principal-Components Analysis

An examination of the complete criterion-referenced data set gathered at Time 1 show that many of the variables are correlated. As discussed in Section 6.6.3, variables within domains are often highly inter-correlated. In addition, some variables in different domains correlate; eg., some of the cognitive variables are correlated with some of the social variables, some fine-motor variables are correlated with independence in activities of daily living variables, etc.

A Principal-Components Analysis of data from 41 functional and physical variables at Time 1 was carried out in order to summarise the relationships between them. The variables are listed in Appendix 6.4. Ten factors were identified after varimax rotation and Kaiser normalisation (Table 6.14), seven of which show interpretable patterns of association (Table 6.15) and are described below. On the other hand, Factor 3 does not show a coherent pattern of association between variables, only Height and Weight variables load on Factor 7 which is, therefore, not particularly interesting, while Two-Hand Coordination of the Fine-Motor Assessment and Attention and Control of Adaptive Behaviour load on Factor 9 and this is not a useful association between variables.

6.6.4.1   Factor 1 (Gross-Motor)

The following variables load heavily on Factor 1; Physical scale of Developmental Profile II, Gross-Motor Scale of Adaptive Behaviour, seven of the nine variables from the direct assessment of gross-motor functioning. Factor 1 can, therefore, be thought of as a 'gross-motor' factor.

6.6.4.2   Factor 2 (Expressive Language)

Factor 2 can be termed 'expressive language' because the following variables have high loadings; Communication scale of Developmental Profile II and six variables from the Language Assessment, namely, Motor Control 1, Motor Control 2, Motor Control 3, Expressive Non-Verbal, Articulation, Expressive Verbal.

6.6.4.3   Factor 4 (Cognitive and Social)

The following variables load heavily on Factor 4; Academic and Social scales of Developmental Profile II, General Cognition scale of Pictorial Test of Intelligence, Interpersonal, Play, Attention and Control scales of Adaptive Behaviour. Factor 4 can, therefore, be called a 'cognitive and social' factor.

6.6.4.4   Factor 5 (Independence and Motor)

Factor 5 can be termed 'independence and motor' because four of the Fine-Motor scales (Independence, Object Transfer 1, Object Transfer 2, Manipulation), Neurology scale, Gross-Motor and Activities of Daily Living scales of Adaptive Behaviour load heavily.

6.6.4.5   Factor 6 (Physical and Gross-Motor)

The following variables load heavily on Factor 6; three of the Gross-Motor scales (Postural Independence, Position Changing Independence, Position Changing Rate) and two of the Physical scales (Hip Mobility, Hamstring, Extensibility). This factor is, therefore, a 'physical and gross-motor' factor.

6.6.4.6   Factor 8 (Behaviour Problems)

One variable has a very high loading on Factor 8 to the exclusion of all others; namely Behaviour Problems. It is, perhaps, interesting that the number of behavioural problems manifested by individual children is not related highly to any other functional variable.

6.6.4.7   Factor 10 (Independence and Social)

Only one variable loads heavily on Factor 10, namely, Self-Help scale of Developmental Profile II, while the Academic and Social scales of

Developmental Profile II load less heavily. This factor can be termed an 'independence and social' factor.

6.6.5 Data Reduction

The results of a principal-components analysis of Time 1 criterion-referenced data suggested a way of taking account of the pattern of correlations between the many variables, for the calculation of seven global scores which provided a summary of each child's functioning, ie., scores for the gross-motor factor, expressive language factor, cognitive and social factor, independence and motor factor, physical and gross-motor factor, behaviour problems factor, and independence and social factor.

As a first step, all test scores were converted to a uniform scale so that scores from different tests could be combined; ie., for a particular test, the mean and standard deviation for the group of 35 children at Time 1 was used to convert an individual's Time 1 and Time 3 test score into two Z scores. If a child improved relative to the Time 1 group mean, the signed Z score increased at Time 3. If a child did not improve or fell behind the initial group mean, the signed Z score remained unchanged or decreased, respectively. Time 2 Z scores were not calculated because the Time 2 assessments did not include a gross-motor assessment or physical assessment, hence, data reduction was not possible.

The next step in obtaining a factor score for each child on, for example, the gross-motor factor at Time 1, was to multiply a child's Time 1 Z score for the eight high loading variables (Table 6.15) by the loading (rounded to one decimal place) then summing these eight weighted Z scores. Similarly, a factor score for Time 3 for the gross-motor factor was obtained by multiplying the Time 3 Z scores for the same eight high loading variables by the loading, before summing the weighted Z scores. A similar procedure was followed to obtain scores for the other six factors at Time 1 and Time 3. These summary data are reported and analysed in Section 6.8.3.

6.7 COMPARISON BETWEEN THE BIRMINGHAM AND MANCHESTER GROUPS ON COLLATERAL DATA

6.7.1 Introduction

The development of the Birmingham and Manchester groups was compared on functional and physical variables (Sections 6.2, 6.8). The interpretation of the results of this comparison required a range of what is to be termed 'collateral data' for three reasons.

113

First, it was not possible to assign children randomly to the two groups and the research team had no control over the selection of the Birmingham group. The initial stages of recruitment in Birmingham involved an element of 'self-selection' because only parents who wanted conductive education for their children responded to the Birmingham Institute's 'Notice of Admission', while later stages involved Hungarian conductors screening and selecting from these 'self-selected' children (Section 6.3). For the selection of a comparison group, it was necessary to go outside the catchment area of the Birmingham Institute. While every effort was made to duplicate the Birmingham procedure in Manchester and to match the two groups closely (Section 6.4), the initial element of 'self-selection' was absent. It was, therefore, necessary to establish whether there were any differences in the backgrounds of the groups which might affect their progress.

Second, the research team had no control over the programmes of education in which the two groups were enrolled. While some differences between conductive education and United Kingdom special education are detailed in Section 3 together with a number of predictions relating to outcome, additional information was gathered on the education timetables and the attendance of the children.

Third, the battery of assessments used for the measurement of children's progress, was designed to yield general functional and physical measures, and not to be specifically relevant to either programme of education. To investigate whether this was achieved, staff involved with the delivery of the programmes were interviewed for their opinion on whether the programmes focused on areas of function assessed by the battery and on possible areas of function not assessed by the battery.

6.7.2 Background of the Groups

6.7.2.1 Educational Experiences Before Time 1 Assessments

Parents were interviewed to get information on educational experiences of the children prior to Time 1 assessments. The age at which a child first became involved in some form of intervention that could be broadly termed 'educational' was established. Such intervention could include contact with an assessment unit, any kind of professionally prescribed home programme including physiotherapy, or enrolment in any kind of school. The two groups do not differ on this variable (Table 6.16).

The period between the first educational intervention and Time 1 assessments was also established and the two groups do not differ (Table 6.16). In other words, the two groups do not differ either with respect to the age at which they first became involved in some form of education or in the period over which the education took place prior to Time 1.

6.7.2.2 Family Background

Information was obtained from questionnaires, supplemented by interviews if necessary, on a range of factors relating to family background. A classification of social class was made on the basis of the father's occupation in two-parent families, or the mother's occupation in one-parent families (Classification of Occupations, 1980). The number of families falling under the following four categories was determined; social class I and II (professional and intermediate occupations), social class III M and III N (skilled manual and skilled non-manual occupations), social class IV and V partly skilled and unskilled occupations), unemployed. Table 6.17 gives the relevant data. A chi squared test was carried out to determine whether the two groups differ significantly in the number of families falling under the three 'employed' categories. It was necessary to combine the social class III M and III N category with the social class IV and V category because of low 'expected' frequencies. The two groups do not differ significantly with respect to the frequency of families falling under the categories of social class I and II and social class III M, III N, IV and V (chi square=0.98).

The two groups are closely matched on frequency of the following; mother's ethnic grouping, 'one-parent' and 'two-parent' families, family size (Table 6.18).

6.7.2.3 Factors Relating to the Mothers During the Evaluation

Questionnaires were sent out to each mother at Time 1, Time 2 and Time 3 seeking information on her psychological well-being, her feelings about the help received by her child and her feelings about the progress made by her child.

Each mother completed a Malaise Inventory (Appendix 6.5) consisting of 24 items relating to backache, feelings of tiredness, depression, headache, irritability, indigestion, etc. Each item was scored 0 or 1 depending on whether the mother does or does not experience the problem behaviour described and the maximum score of 24 indicates a good state of psychological well-being. Mean scores and standard deviations for the two groups at Time 1, Time 2 and Time 3 are given in Table 6.19. Each mother also indicated on a nine-point scale what she felt about her life as a whole, the help her child is receiving and the progress being made by her child (Appendix 6.6). Mean scores and standard deviations for the two groups at Time 1, Time 2 and Time 3 are given in Table 6.19. Occasionally, some mothers did not return their questionnaires and this accounts for the small change in the size of the groups.

Two-way analyses of variance (Group × Time) yielded only one significant result; the Group effect was significant for 'mother's satisfaction with help received by child', with the Birmingham mothers indicating greater satisfaction than the Manchester mothers (F (1,31) 69.71, p < .01). No other Group effects were significant and none of the Time effects or Group × Time interactions were significant.

The data show that the mothers gave similar scores at Time 1, Time 2 and Time 3 on each variable and the groups were closely matched on mothers' psychological well-being and mothers' feeling about life as a whole. On the other hand, while mothers of the Birmingham group rated the help received by their children more highly than mothers of the Manchester group, the groups were closely matched on mothers' feeling about their childrens' progress.

Related data were gathered as part of the work to be described in Section 6.7.2.4. Some mothers found it difficult to respond to questions in the questionnaire, eg., it was difficult for a mother to indicate on the nine-point scale what she felt about the progress made by her child when there was high satisfaction with some aspects of progress but low satisfaction with others.

In order to provide a perhaps more accurate picture of 'satisfaction with progress', the social worker, during the interview with parents at Time 2 and Time 3, asked the parents how they felt generally about their child's progress over the previous year at the Institute or at the relevant school. The response of the parents was categorised as follows: generally very satisfied, generally satisfied, mixed (progress better in some areas than others), generally not satisfied. The number of families in each category of response is shown in Table 6.20.

Time 1—Time 2.   While some parents in both groups who expressed themselves as 'very satisfied' used words such as 'brilliant', 'marvellous', 'smashing', 'amazing' and 'fantastic' to emphasize their point, overall, the Birmingham parents tended to be less qualified in their responses than the Manchester parents. This can be illustrated as follows:

All the Birmingham parents declared themselves 'very satisfied' or 'satisfied' though there were a few reservations. Eight parents expressed mild dissatisfaction with academic or 'school work' aspects, though four of these thought that while the children were missing out on this at present, it was likely that they would catch up later. One family was concerned about the child's frequent falls at the Institute. Another family was concerned about the process of decision making about when a child should leave the Institute.

While ten Manchester parents were unreserved in declaring themselves 'very satisfied', the two parents who were 'satisfied', qualified their statements. Furthermore, unlike the Birmingham group, there were two parents in the 'mixed' category (clearly differentiating between aspects of their child's development), and three parents in the 'not satisfied' category who also explained why ('very slow—no improvement in walking', 'hasn't come on much—not pushed enough', 'were satisfied but less so since the change of teacher').

Time 2—Time 3. Over the second period of the evaluation, the Birmingham parents showed a clear fall in 'satisfaction with progress' while the Manchester parents showed a modest improvement. This can be illustrated as follows:

The number of Birmingham parents saying they were 'very satisfied' dropped from 16 to 6, a decline borne out by the less enthusiastic language used by parents in responding to this question than in the first period. Among the nine parents in the 'satisfied' category, comments were made that progress was less impressive than in the first period, while there were now four parents in the 'mixed' category, all of whom were pleased with their children's physical progress but not so pleased with educational or other aspects of development.

In contrast, the Manchester group showed a slight overall increase in 'satisfaction with progress' at the lower end of the scale, with no parents declaring themselves 'not satisfied'. Parents in the 'mixed' category were pleased with most aspects of development *except* walking and mobility—the reverse of the Birmingham situation.

In summary, there seems to be a curious inconsistency in the mother's view of the help received by their children and their view of the children's progress. The Birmingham mothers gave higher scores than the Manchester mothers on a scale relating to the help received by their children, which indicates an appreciation in the Birmingham mothers of the time and effort expended by staff of the Institute on the children. However, the Birmingham mothers did not register an additional 'pay-off' in terms of development because they did not give higher scores than the Manchester mothers on a scale relating to the progress made by their children; rather, the two groups of mothers gave similar scores on this scale. Furthermore, there seemed to be a fall over time in 'satisfaction with progress' among the Birmingham parents but not among the Manchester parents.

6.7.2.4 Out-of-School Factors Possibly Affecting Function

6.7.2.4.1 *Introduction*

All children in both groups continued to live at home with their families and attend the Institute or their schools on a daily basis with the normal school holidays. It was considered possible that measures of their progress might be affected by input or circumstances originating outside the education programmes. It is not unusual for children, whether in mainstream or special education, to receive special help or attention outside school (tuition in academic subjects, development of special talents, social and recreational opportunities, etc), while their progress and development may also be affected by illness, medical, surgical or therapeutic treatment, or a variety of more or less traumatic family circumstances or changes.

The Birmingham group was 'self-selected' in the first stage of enrolment at the Institute and it was necessary for parents to make an effort in seeking alternative education for their children. It is, therefore, feasible that these parents might be more motivated in helping their children compared to parents of the Manchester group who followed the conventional course of enrolling their children in the local special school. Greater motivation might be translated into greater effort in helping the children and also in protecting them from factors that might have an adverse effect on their development. It seemed necessary to investigate the out-of-school lives of the two groups and to establish whether there were any overall differences in factors that could possibly affect function. If differences were found, they would need to be taken into account in evaluating any differences between the groups in their development. If not, differences in the development of the groups could be ascribed to differences between their education programmes.

Interviews with parents of all children were carried out by a social worker with considerable experience of working with children and their families. The aim was as follows; to establish whether there were any major differences between the groups in factors operating outside the education programmes which might have a bearing on the development of the children. Two broad classes of developmental variables were to be considered; variables which were being assessed by the researchers and variables which were not being assessed but might be important in a child's overall development. In practice, the assessments carried out by the researchers covered such a broad range of variables that parents rarely mentioned an aspect of development which could not be considered relevant to a research variable. A schedule was needed to guide the interviewer in a systematic enquiry while allowing the parents some freedom to discuss the child's development.

6.7.2.4.2 Categories of Input

The main concern had been to check whether or not the children were experiencing out-of-school programmes or input of a planned or organised nature which might be beneficial to their functioning and also to take into account anything that might have held them back. Such programmes or interventions, it was surmised, might be provided by professionals from a variety of disciplines, by parents, other family members or friends, or by voluntary or statutory services or groups.

Four categories of input were envisaged: 1. family input; 2. input from educational and paramedical professionals such as teachers, physiotherapists, occupational therapists and speech therapists; 3. input from medical professionals including surgery; 4. other input or circumstances not fitting into the previous three categories.

Family input was to include any activity with the child which, in the parent's estimation, resulted in some difference in the child's functioning. Such input, whether in the form of planned programmes or informal activities would be likely to be present in every family to some degree and the interviewer would need to bear in mind some qualifications.

First, many activities likely to be reported by parents, would not differ from those frequently undertaken by parents with non-handicapped children, and indeed, would often be considered 'normal' in bringing up children. However, when one considers the special degree of effort and patience required in order to teach many children with cerebral palsy simple everyday skills, the significance of the family input becomes clearer. Washing, toileting, dressing, for example, need reserves of patience, perseverance and encouragement to help children towards independence, while normally enjoyable activities like walks in the park, swimming, conversation may require time and commitment not generally demanded of parents.

Second, the activities or occurrences recorded would be those which the parents chose to mention to the interviewer in response to a consistent series of exploratory questons; eg., 'What usually happens with . . . when he/she returns home after school/at weekends/during holidays?' Similarly, it would be the parents' view of the effect of these activities on the children which would be recorded; the interviewer's observation of family interacton or the child's behaviour might in some cases be a useful supplement, but the judgments would essentially be subjective.

Input under the second and third category listed above would be somewhat easier to establish than 'family input', because formal contact with professionals would be required and the types of programmes or intervention would be specific for children with cerebral palsy.

The last category of input could not be entirely predicted, but was expected to include, for example, illness, family changes, alternative care arrangements, statutory or voluntary group activities.

6.7.2.4.3 *Areas of Function*

Section 6.2 reports the assessments which were carried out on the children by the researchers. It was necessary to provide the social worker with a listing of the types of functions which were being assessed so that she could categorise parents' responses to interview questions.

The task of listing the types of functions assessed by the researchers was not straight forward. Some assessments cover a wide range of different types of functions and the raw scores reflect a diverse set of abilities. For example, the Physical Scale of Developmental Profile II has items covering a wide range of fine-motor and gross-motor activities, while the Vineland Adaptive Behaviour Personal Subdomain includes items concerned with eating, dressing, toileting and bathing. It would be impractical to try and establish how factors at home, for example, would bear on one of these scales when so many different types of functions are grouped together.

On the other hand, there is considerable overlap between different parts of the assessment. For example, there are items dealing with mathematical skills in the Achievement Assessment, Pictorial Test of Intelligence and three scales of Developmental Profile II. As another example, there are items dealing with crawling in the Gross Motor Assessment, Vineland Adaptive Behaviour Gross Motor Subdomain, and the Physical Scale of Developmental Profile II. Clearly items of similar type needed to be identified and grouped together.

The contents of all the assessments were therefore listed in detail (840 items) and then grouped into 53 categories of function. The categories themselves were then grouped under seven main headings: namely, mental functioning, communication, fine-motor functioning, gross-motor functioning, personal behaviour, interpersonal behaviour, self-help behaviour. This proved a manageable framework for analysing the responses of parents to the interview questions.

Appendix 6.7 lists the 53 categories of function under the seven main headings. Under each category there is a listing of the type of individual assessment items.

6.7.2.4.4 General Form of the Interview

Each interview had the same general form outlined in Appendix 6.8. The success of these family interviews in eliciting informaton which might include sensitive material about family matters and previously undeclared help for the children, was likely to depend on the establishment of a good rapport between the interviewer and the parents as well as parental confidence that information given would not be misused or work to the detriment of the child. These requirements had certain implications for the structure of the interview.

First, parents were assured that information would be kept confidential to the research team and that no child or family would be identified in any published report.

Second, the interview was structured but not formal or rigid. The interviewer asked consistent questions but followed up parental replies in a flexible way and did not 'tick off' a lengthy series of categories and sub-categories of the assessment schedule as if filling in a questionnaire. This was particularly relevant to exploring 'family input'. In order to gain information about the general nature of parent-child interaction without asking leading questions, parents were asked what happened during the period between coming home from school and bedtime, and also during weekends and holiday periods. They were then asked about any activities they mentioned to establish the effect of these activities on their child's functioning.

Third, it was considered desirable to interview parents at home, because of the likely convenience for them, their increased confidence in being on 'home ground', the opportunity to include both parents (where relevant) and to glimpse family functioning at first hand. The parents were, however, offered a choice of venue, eg., the school.

Fourth, notes were made of responses to questions and other comments during the interview (Appendix 6.9) and the resulting information was later encoded on a data sheet (Appendix 6.9).

6.7.2.4.5 *Encoding of Data*

The aim of the interview was for the social worker to complete a data sheet for each child (Appendix 6.9). For example, if during the course of the interview the parent said that a member of the family often helped the child to read at home, an entry would be made under family input (Input 1) against the 'cognitive functioning' category because the ability to read is assessed by the research team and the assessment is included under the main category of cognitive functioning (Appendix 6.7). As another example, if the child received help from a speech therapist at home to communicate non-verbally through a system of symbols and signs, an entry would be made under speech therapy (Input 2) against the 'communication' category because the ability to communicate nonverbally is assessed and the assessment is included under the main category of communication (Appendix 6.7).

Discussion of how the effect of any input should be judged and recorded led to the conclusion that it could only be, in the main, by the parents' own view on whether it had, overall, helped or hindered their child's development. Such views would, of course, be subjective and lacking any measurement, but only if there were noticeable differences between the two groups in input and outcomes for the children, might it be necessary to look more closely into what had been happening.

A single input could be entered against more than one area of function if it was the parent's view that the input affected functions in more than one area; eg., surgical intervention might be considered to have affected several different assessed functions like 'gross-motor' (mobility) 'cognitive' (absence from school) and 'self-help behaviour' (toileting, dressing, etc).

6.7.2.4.6   Timing of Interviews

The plan was to carry out interviews to coincide with Time 2 and Time 3 assessments for the Birmingham and Manchester groups and parents were questioned about possible out-of-school factors affecting their children during the previous year; ie., Time 1—Time 2 period and Time 2—Time 3 period (Section 6.3.5 and Section 6.4.3). There were difficulties in funding this part of the evaluation and the Time 2 interviews for the Birmingham group could not begin until September 1990. Other interviews were carried out closer to schedule. In all cases, however, the interviewer clarified the period being discussed and assisted the parents by encouraging them to think back over the year's landmarks (Christmas, holiday times, birthdays, etc), to recall events or circumstances, or to check diaries if these were used. A total of 19 Birmingham parents and 20 Manchester parents were interviewed although data from only 17 of the latter will be reported (Section 6.5).

6.7.2.4.7   Letters to Parents

A letter was sent out to all parents to introduce the interviewer who subsequently made contact to set an appointment and explain the purpose of the interviews (Appendix 6.10).

6.7.2.4.8   Preparation for Interviews

For both groups, the interviewer visited the Institute or the special schools before visiting the families. These visits had two purposes: to gain some idea from staff about the facilities, programmes and general organisation of the children's school life, and to observe the children in the course of their normal activities in order to recognise them as individuals and observe how they functioned in school. These visits were very useful for the interviewer in understanding the educational context of the children's lives and later, sharing that understanding with their families.

6.7.2.4.9   Results

Table 6.21 gives the number of times parents in the Birmingham (N=19) and Manchester (N=17) groups reported input under four categories (1. family input, 2. input from educational and paramedical professionals, 3. input from medical professionals, 4. other input) having helpful, hindering and uncertain effects on seven areas of function assessed by the research team (cognition, communication, fine-motor, gross-motor, personal, inter-personal, self-help) during the period between Time 1 and Time 2 assessments. Table 6.22 gives the relevant data for the period between Time 2 and Time 3 assessments. The totals at the bottom of Tables 6.21

and 6.22 show that over both periods, parents reported most input under the 'family input' category and the effect of this input was generally considered to be helpful. Of the total number of inputs reported by the Birmingham and Manchester parents, 76 per cent was under the 'helpful family input' category in the Time 1—Time 2 period while 80 per cent came under this category in the Time 2—Time 3 period. Given the low incidence of report in the other eleven categories, the statistical comparison between the groups will be limited to the 'helpful family input' category.

Table 6.23 gives the means and standard deviations for the two groups in the incidence of family input reported by parents as 'helpful' to areas of function assessed by the research team over the Time 1—Time 2 and Time 2—Time 3 periods, including input summed over all areas of function. An analysis of variance showed that the groups did not differ and there was no change over time in either group in the overall incidence of 'helpful family input'.

The means in Table 6.23 conceal wide variations between families in their reported incidence of 'helpful family input'; eg., for the Time 1—Time 2 period, the lowest and highest reported total incidence was 5 and 19 respectively. In looking for family characteristics which might be associated with this variation, the relationship with social class (Section 6.7.2.2) was investigated. Leaving aside families in the 'unemployed' category, the correlations between social class and incidence of 'helpful family input' for the Time 1—Time 2 period was as follows: Birmingham, $r_s=0.07$, N=14, NS; Manchester $r_s=0.60$, N=13, p < .05. The result for Manchester is, perhaps, what one might expect intuitively; ie., the higher the family's social class, the higher its reported incidence of 'helpful family input'. The lack of such a relationship in Birmingham may reflect the element of 'self-selection' in the recruitment of the children (Section 6.7.1). Across the range of social class, parents in Birmingham were actively seeking alternative education for their children, hence the, perhaps, expected relationship between social class and helpful family input is masked in the Birmingham group by homogeneity among the parents in their determination to help their children.

6.7.3   Education Programmes

Differences between conductive education and United Kingdom special education are described in Section 3 and three predictions were made regarding the relative efficacy of the two systems in promoting the development of children with cerebral palsy. The description and the predictions were based on information gathered from direct observation of the programmes and from discussions with staff involved with the delivery of the programmes. This was later supplemented by a comparison between the groups with respect to the destination of the children during the evaluation, attendance by the children in their programmes and also by an attempt to compare the programmes with respect to the timetable followed by the children. The following sections report these supplementary data.

6.7.3.1   Destination of the Children During the Evaluation

It had always been anticipated that children might be discharged from the Birmingham Institute or from one of the schools in Manchester during the period of the evaluation. There was also a possibility that children might regularly attend another school part-time especially in Manchester where there is a policy in one of the schools of having children enrolled in mainstream schools for part of each school day as a preparation for full-time enrolment. In either event, the assessment of the children would continue as scheduled, provided the parents continued to consent to involvement with the evaluation. Any benefits experienced by the children during their time in conductive education or their time in the Manchester programmes, might be expected to transfer to the new educational setting. For the present purpose, a child was considered as being discharged into another programme if enrolled full-time or part-time at another school during the Time 1—Time 2 or Time 2—Time 3 periods.

Data in Table 6.24 show that a total of four children were discharged from the Birmingham Institute into mainstream schools during the period of the evaluation. Another two children went to a special school; one child was withdrawn from the Institute by the parents while the other child was discharged by the conductors because they felt the child had progressed as far as possible in the only group available in Birmingham (Section 4.8). A total of five children were discharged from the Manchester schools into mainstream schools, while no child went to another special school. It can, therefore, be concluded that there was no major difference between the groups with respect to change in educational experiences during the period of the evaluation.

6.7.3.2   Attendance by the Children

Assessments of the children in both groups were carried out, nominally, at the beginning of each calendar year (Section 6.3.5 and Section 6.4.4). The period between assessments therefore spanned academic years; eg., a new academic year began in Manchester in September 1990, hence, the period between the Time 1 assessment (1 January 1990) and the Time 2 assessment (1 January 1991) included the second part of the 1989/90 and the first part of the 1990/91 academic years. The number of half-days a programme of education was open to each child in both groups during the calendar year between consecutive assessments was recorded from the relevant school registers. Half-days involving outside events organized by the school or outside programmes agreed by the school were included. If a child changed schools during the calendar year, the registers of both schools were consulted. Data reported in Table 6.25 give the wrong impression that some schools may have failed to provide the statutory minimum requirement of 190 full days of education in each academic year. The totals sometimes fall short of 190 full days because the data come from the second part of one academic year and the first part of the following academic year and the number of days of education available before and after the New Year varies between academic years.

The number of half-days each child was absent from the available programme of education was also recorded and expressed as a percentage of the available number of half-days of education.

Data in Table 6.25 show that the Birmingham group had more days of education available in each 12 month period than the Manchester group. On the other hand, a two-way analysis of variance on 'percentage absenteeism' (Group × Time) yielded non-significant results, showing that absenteeism was similar in the two groups over the period of the evaluation.

6.7.3.3 Timetables

It was beyond the resources of the research team to maintain a continuous record of the timetables followed by the children in the two groups. This would have been especially difficult for the Manchester group where each child had an individual timetable which might change at various times during the year. It was decided, therefore, to document the timetable followed by each child in a single week in the period between the Time 2 and Time 3 assessments. This would give an indication of differences between individual children within a group although there would be no data on variations in the timetable throughout the year. One child in each group was transferred to a mainstream school between Time 1 and Time 2 and they are not included here (Table 6.24). In the case of children transferred to alternative education between Time 2 and Time 3 (Table 6.24), data were gathered only with respect to the timetable followed prior to the children being transferred.

During the planning stage of this part of the evaluation, it became clear that it would be difficult to design a strictly quantitative comparison between the Birmingham and Manchester programmes; ie., directly comparing the two programmes on the amount of time spent on educating various aspects of cognitive, communication, motor, social and independence functioning. The two programmes would differ qualitatively not just quantitatively in having different curricula, with children being taught a particular topic or skill in one programme but not in the other, eg., being taught a system of 'signing' as a means of non-verbal communication in Manchester but not in Birmingham. Even where the programmes shared a common curriculum, it would be incorrect to assume that two classes with the same title shared equivalent teaching methods and aims, eg., a 'walking' programme in Birmingham involves different physical aids to a 'walking' programme in Manchester and the programmes do not share exactly the same aim in promoting a child's mobility. There are further problems in so far as a given programme may involve multiple activities and have multiple objectives in Birmingham, while a programme with a similar title in Manchester may be more focused, so making any direct comparison difficult; eg., a 'walking' programme in Birmingham involves much singing and reciting with the aim of facilitating both walking and the development of speech, while a 'walking' programme in Manchester may focus only on the activity of walking with singing being taught in a separate period of the day. It was decided, therefore, not to compare the two programmes on the details of particular topics or skills which are taught, but rather aim for a comparison based on a broad categorisation of topics and skills.

Staff involved with the education of the children first provided the timetable followed by each child during the chosen week. This was done partly by the staff filling out a pre-prepared form and partly by interview during which staff and a member of the research team clarified the objectives of the exercise and the meaning of the staffs' responses. The length of each formal period in the day was required together with a general description of the lesson or programme rather than a precise account of the content.

A major difference between the programmes became immediately apparent. The timetable in Birmingham was very quickly documented because staff indicated that all the children were engaged in a single timetabled programme. In contrast, much effort was required to document the programme in Manchester because each child followed a different timetable and separate interviews were required even for children within one school.

An attempt was made to allocate each period of the day into one of five categories according to the main objective of the programme or lesson and the nature of the activity involved; academic, physical, life skills, social, arts. These categories were to include periods with the following general description:

Academic	Pre-maths, maths, pre-reading, reading, story telling, writing, science, technology, computers.
Physical	Any form of lying, sitting, standing, walking, mobility or hand function programme as well as physiotherapy, occupational therapy, speech therapy and swimming.
Life Skills	Toileting, dressing, cookery, use of library, learning about the 'outside' world.
Social	Assembly, news, TV, role-play, structured play, games.
Arts	Crafts, construction toys, drama, moving to music, singing.

It became apparent, however, that even a five-way categorisation as broad as this was effectively impossible for the Birmingham group because all periods involve multiple objectives. For example, a sitting programme would certainly belong in the 'physical' category because of the gross motor action of sitting and because it involves speech, but it would also belong in the 'social' category because the development of interpersonal relationships is encouraged and the 'arts' category because the children can be required to sing. As another example, children are required to walk outdoors in order to examine a plant in the garden. Such a programme would belong in the 'physical' category because of the walking but also the 'academic' category because the examination of the plant may be part of a science programme and the 'life skills' category because the children must learn to walk in contexts outside the Institute. Different periods place different emphases on the various categories and it is impractical to attempt to 'parcel-out' the week's programme into periods of time spent on each of the categories of topics and skills being taught.

Despite the difficulties, however, and putting aside the issue of content, an overall examination of the timetables seemed to suggest marked differences between Birmingham and Manchester in the amount of time spent on programmes of a primarily 'academic' nature and programmes primarily involved with improving skills which demand gross-motor functioning, fine-motor functioning and functioning of the speech apparatus ('physical' programmes).

Considering the 'physical' category first, the Birmingham children were each engaged for a total of 14.0 hours per week in the following types of clearly physical programmes; 'lying' (3.5 hours), 'standing and walking' (2.5 hours), 'walking' (4.0 hours), 'sitting' (3.0 hours), 'speech' (1.0 hours). There were other programmes which placed a heavy demand on motor functioning like handwriting, dressing and feeding, but these are not included in the above tally because they had clear concurrent objectives.

In the case of the Manchester children, the number of hours spent in physiotherapy, speech therapy, occupational therapy, swimming, physical education and any other programme specifically aimed at improving fine-motor functioning, gross-motor functioning and speech was tallied. As with Birmingham, any programme which placed a heavy demand on motor functioning but with additional objectives was not included. The average number of hours spent per week on 'physical' programmes was 3.3 hours (25 per cent of the time spent by Birmingham children) and there were wide variations among the children from as little as 1 hour per week to a maximum of 4.5 hours per week.

Considering now the 'academic' category, the Birmingham children were each engaged for a total of 4.0 hours per week in the following types of programmes; maths (2.0 hours), reading and writing (2.0 hours).

The Manchester children, on average, spent a similar amount of time to the Birmingham children on maths, reading and writing, but they were also engaged in a wide range of other programmes of a clearly 'academic' nature including science, technology and 'topic work'. The average number of hours spent per week on 'academic' programmes was 8.0 hours (double the time spent by Birmingham children) and there were variations among the children ranging from as little as 4.0 hours per week, to a maximum of 11.8 hours per week.

Finally, it can be noted that while many special schools in the United Kingdom have periods of the day scheduled for conductive education type programmes which include activities modelled on so-called 'task series' (Section 5.4.2.2), children in the Manchester group were not engaged in such programmes in their schools during the period of the study. Only one child in the Manchester group was exposed to a conductive education type of programme external to the school and this was part-time on a small scale during the Time 2—Time 3 period. This child's exposure to conductive education was negligible compared to that of children in the Birmingham group.

In summary, this attempt to document and compare the timetables followed by the two groups of children indicates the following (see also Section 3.7):

First, while there was virtually no variability in the timetable followed by the Birmingham group, each child in the Manchester group had an individual timetable.

Second, the Birmingham timetable had a four-fold longer amount of time allocated to programmes of a clearly physical nature but half the time allocated to programmes of a clearly academic nature compared to the Manchester timetable.

Third, the Manchester children were virtually free of exposure to conductive education.

6.7.4   Relevance of the Research Assessments to the Programmes of Education

6.7.4.1   Introduction

While the battery of assessments used for the measurement of children's progress was tailored neither to conductive education nor to United Kingdom education, an attempt was made to confirm whether bias in the relevance of the battery to the specific programmes had been avoided. Staff involved with the delivery of the programmes were interviewed for their opinion on the extent to which the programmes focused on areas of function assessed by the battery and on other possible areas not assessed by the battery. Any major differences between the groups in the staff's perception of the relevance of the assessments to the programmes, would help in interpreting possible differences between the groups in how they progressed on the assessments.

6.7.4.2   Areas of Function

Section 6.7.2.4.3 describes how the types of functions assessed by the researchers were listed for the interview concerning out-of-school factors which may have affected the functioning of the children. Appendix 6.7 lists 53 categories of function under seven main headings together with the range of individual assessment items included under each category. The same listing was used for the present interview.

6.7.4.3   General Form of the Interview

A member of the research team carried out interviews with members of staff involved with the delivery of the programmes. In Birmingham there was one interviewee for all the children, namely, the senior Hungarian conductor seconded from the Pető Institute as the group leader. In Manchester, class teachers and physiotherapists who were responsible for the children's programmes were interviewed. For both groups, interviews were carried out after the Time 2 assessment and were meant to cover programmes delivered in the period between Time 1 and Time 2 assessments (Section 6.3.5, Section 6.4.4). An interview was not carried out for one of the children in the Birmingham group because the child was discharged from the Institute before the Time 2 assessment (Section 6.7.3.1). The data to be reported are, therefore, based on 18 children in Birmingham and 17 children in Manchester.

The purpose of the interview was explained in the following terms; to obtain the staff's view on whether areas of function assessed by the research team were foci of the programmes and whether there were any other areas of function focused on by the programmes which were not assessed for the research. The purpose was *not* to document the needs of the children or whether the programmes on offer were effective.

The interviewer was provided with a set of data sheets for each child similar to that given in Appendix 6.11, which listed the 53 categories of function under the following seven headings; 'mental functioning', 'communication', 'fine-motor functioning', 'gross-motor functioning', 'personal behaviour', 'interpersonal behaviour' and 'self-help behaviour'. The interviewer also had a listing of the types of assessment items included under the 53 categories (Appendix 6.7). There was space provided on each data sheet for the entry of categories of function which the staff said were foci of the programmes but which could not be placed under any of the research headings.

The interviews were semi-structured, the list of functions under the seven headings were discussed and each function was given a 'relevance' score of 0, 1, 2 or 3 if, in the staff's opinion, the function was not a focus, a minor focus, a medium focus or a major focus of the programme, respectively, over the previous year. Any extra categories to be included in the list were to be scored on a similar scale.

6.7.4.4 Results

The list of functions assessed by the research staff was sufficiently broad to cover all foci of the Birmingham and Manchester programmes—staff in neither group mentioned foci which were outside the listing of research assessments provided for the interview (Appendix 6.11, Appendix 6.7).

'Relevance' scores for categories of function under each functional heading were summed for each child and the group means and standard deviations are given in Table 6.26. Staff in Birmingham and Manchester differed in their opinion about the relevance of the research assessments to the programmes of education; ie., it was thought that conductive education focused significantly more on functions assessed under the headings of 'fine-motor functioning', 'gross-motor functioning' and 'self-help behaviour' than the programmes in Manchester. Conversely, while staff in Manchester tended to give functions under the headings of 'communication' and 'interpersonal behaviour' higher 'relevance' scores than in Birmingham, the difference was not statistically significant.

The particular categories of function receiving higher 'relevance' scores in Birmingham than in Manchester were as follows:

Fine-motor functioning; 'grasping, placing, releasing objects', 'differentiated control of fingers', 'two-hand coordination', 'use of pencil and paper', 'throwing and catching'.

Gross-motor functioning; 'static postures', 'position changing', 'crawling, creeping', 'walking without aids'.

Self-help behaviour; 'drinking', 'eating', 'dressing, undressing', 'toileting', 'washing, drying', 'grooming'.

Finally, the standard deviations in Table 6.25 suggest that there was greater variability among the Manchester children in the relevance of the research assessments than among the Birmingham children; ie., the foci of programmes in Manchester tended to vary more from child to child than the foci of programmes in Birmingham. This supports an observation made in Section 6.7.3.3 that children in Birmingham were engaged in a single timetabled programme, while children in Manchester had more individualised programmes.

6.7.5   Conclusions

As outlined in Section 6.7.1, it was necessary to compare the Birmingham and Manchester groups on a range of collateral data in order to interpret possible differences in their development. Three sets of conclusions can be made.

First, the initial stages of recruitment in Birmingham involved an element of 'self-selection' that was absent in Manchester and it was, therefore, necessary to establish whether there were any differences between the groups in background and family circumstances which might affect their progress. Data show that there is no difference between the groups in the age at which the children first experienced some form of 'educational' intervention or the period over which such education took place prior to Time 1 assessments. The two groups were simiar with respect to social class, ethnic grouping, mother's marital status and family size at Time 1. There was no difference between the groups over the period of the evaluation in mothers' psychological well-being, mothers' feeling about life as a whole, or in out-of-school factors like planned programmes or informal activities in the family setting which might have affected the childrens' functioning. It can be concluded, therefore, that there is no evidence that 'self-selection' in Birmingham yielded a group of children with different backgrounds or family circumstances to the Manchester group.

Second, differences between conductive education and United Kingdom special education outlined in Section 3 led to three predictions regarding the superior effectiveness of conductive education (Section 3.7). Data relevant to these predictions reviewed in the present sections show that the groups did not differ with respect to change in educational experiences during the period of the evaluation and absenteeism was similar for the two groups. On the other hand, a range of findings increase the likelihood of Prediction 1 being supported. The Birmingham programme covered more days in the year and involved longer days of work than the Manchester programme (Section 3.6). The Birmingham children were engaged in programmes of a clearly physical nature for a four-fold longer period of time in a week than the Manchester children. Mothers of the Birmingham children scored the help received by their children more highly than mothers of the Manchester children. The likelihood of finding support for Prediction 2 is increased by the indication of less variability among the Birmingham children in their programme compared to the Manchester children.

Third, while the battery of assessments used for the measurement of children's progress was not designed to be specifically relevant to either programme of education, in the opinion of staff involved with the delivery of the programmes, the Birmingham programme focused significantly more intensively on functions assessed by the research team under the headings of fine-motor functioning, gross-motor functioning and self-help behaviour than the Manchester programme. Although this opinion was not investigated further, it does increase the likelihood of finding support for Prediction 1.

6.8 LONGITUDINAL COMPARISON BETWEEN THE BIRMINGHAM AND MANCHESTER GROUPS ON FUNCTIONAL AND PHYSICAL VARIABLES: DISCUSSION OF RESULTS IN RELATION TO COLLATERAL DATA

6.8.1 Introduction

Section 6.2 describes the battery of assessments used for measuring the functional and physical characteristics of children in the Birmingham and Manchester groups, and Section 6.3.5 and Section 6.4.4 give the timing of the assessments. The present section reports comparisons between the groups at Time 1, Time 2 and Time 3 as tests of the predictions relating to the superior effectiveness of conductive education given in Section 3.7. The groups are compared in their development, first on criterion-referenced data, second on Factor scores based on criterion-referenced data, third on variability in criterion-referenced data and fourth on norm-referenced data. Results are discussed in relation to collateral data reported in Section 6.7.

6.8.2 Criterion-Referenced Data

Figures 6.1–6.47 give the results of 47 criterion-referenced variables in the order described in Section 6.2. All the figures have a similar form. In brackets at the top, is the number of the section which describes the variable. The data are plotted and the figures in brackets on the ordinate give the possible range in the criterion-referenced raw score. There is a table giving the size (N), mean and standard deviation (SD) of the Birmingham and Manchester groups at Time 1, Time 2 and Time 3 where data are available. At the bottom is a table summarising the results of a two-way univariate analysis of variance, and t tests are reported comparing Time 1 with Time 2 and Time 2 with Time 3 performance where there are data from these assessments.

6.8.2.1 Group Differences

Only one variable yielded a significant Group effect; ie., Articulation (Figure 6.21). The Birmingham group performed better, overall, on this variable compared to the Manchester group. However, given that the groups do not differ on 46 other variables, the importance of this isolated result is negligible.

132

6.8.2.2 Time Differences

All variables yielded a significant Time effect except Receptive Non-Verbal (Figure 6.18), Pen Placement (Figure 6.28), Hip Mobility (Figure 6.37), Hamstring Extensibility (Figure 6.38) and Behaviour Problems (Figure 6.47). Two of these (Receptive Non-Verbal, Pen Placement) are functional variables which, perhaps, could have been expected to show improvement over time, while two (Hip Mobility and Hamstring Extensibility) are physical variables which might not be expected to change.

An examination of the plots of all the data and the results of 5 tests at the bottom of the figures indicate that some variables show greater improvement between Time 1 and Time 2 than between Time 2 and Time 3. There is, however, only scant evidence for 'ceiling effects' and most Time 3 means are well below the top of the scales. The exceptions are the four parts of the Pre-verbal Communication assessment—Motor Control 3 (Figure 6.17), Receptive Non-Verbal (Figure 6.18), Expressive Non-Verbal (Figure 6.19), Receptive Verbal (Figure 6.20)—as discussed in Section 6.6.2.

In summary, nearly all the functional variables were responsive to changes in the children.

6.8.2.3 Differential Change Over Time

Eight variables showed a significant Group × Time interaction and for six of these, the Manchester group progressed better than the Birmingham group. On Object Transfer 1 (Figure 6.24), Postural Independence (Figure 6.30) and Position Changing Independence (Figure 6.31), the groups had a similar level of performance at Time 1 but the Manchester group subsequently improved more than the Birmingham group. On Form Discrimination (Figure 6.7) and Activities of Daily Living (Figure 6.45), the Manchester group performed worse than the Birmingham group at Time 1 but then improved more and, hence, caught up. On Hip Mobility (Figure 6.37), there was a slight improvement for the Manchester group but a substantial deterioration for the Birmingham group.

On two variables—Interpersonal (Figure 6.43) and Play (Figure 6.44)—the groups showed a different pattern of improvement over time with the Manchester group improving more than the Birmingham group between Time 1 and Time 2, and then the Birmingham group improving more than the Manchester group between Time 2 and Time 3.

In summary, while on most of the 47 functional and physical variables, the two groups showed similar improvement over time, on the few examples where there was a difference in their progress, the difference was in favour of the Manchester group.

6.8.2.4   Discussion (Prediction 1)

Contrary to Prediction 1 (Section 3.7), the only evidence of differences in functional development between children receiving conductive education and children receiving United Kingdom special education is in favour of United Kingdom special education. The Manchester group made better progress than the Birmingham group on one direct test of cognition (Form Discrimination), one direct test of fine-motor functioning (Object Transfer 1), two direct tests of gross-motor functioning (Postural Independence, Position Changing Independence) and one indirect test of independence in daily living skills (Activities of Daily Living). There were no differences between the groups in development on any of the tests of communication or social functioning.

Given the following advantages for the group receiving conductive education compared to the group receiving United Kingdom special education—higher degree of selection and specific grouping of chidren (Section 3.2), longer exposure to the programme in each year (Section 3.6, Section 6.7.3.2), greater exposure to programmes of a clearly physical nature (Section 6.7.3.3), and staff's higher rating to the 'relevance' of the fine-motor, gross-motor and self-help research assessments (Section 6.7.4)—the lack of any evidence of superior rates of progress in the group receiving conductive education can only be interpreted as failure of conductive education in Birmingham to fulfil the high expectations which have come to be associated with this system.

The finding of deterioration in the mobility of the hips in the group receiving conductive education when no such deterioration was seen in the Manchester group may reflect an inadequate consideration in conductive education of the orthopaedic problems of children with cerebral palsy and, for example, the requirement for surgical intervention (Section 2.4, Section 2.5, Section 5.5.3).

6.8.3   Factor Scores Based on Criterion-Referenced Data

Figures 6.48–6.54 give the results of seven Factor scores in the order described in Section 6.6.4. All the figures have a similar form. In brackets at the top is the number of the section which describes the Factor.

The data are plotted and there is a table giving the size (N), mean, and standard deviation (SD) of the Birmingham and Manchester groups at Time 1 and Time 3. At the bottom is a table giving the results of a two-way univariate analysis of variance.

6.8.3.1   Group Differences

The groups do not differ on any of the Factor scores.

6.8.3.2   Time Differences

All Factor scores yielded a significant Time effect, showing that the groups performed better at Time 3 relative to Time 1.

6.8.3.3   Differential Change Over Time

None of the Factor scores yielded a significant Group × Time interaction, indicating that the groups did not differ in the amount of progress over the Time 1 to Time 3 period.

6.8.3.4   Discussion (Prediction 1)

All the Factor scores, calculated for the purpose of summarising the childrens' functioning were responsive to improvement in the children. While the Manchester group tended to show greater progress than the Birmingham group on these global scores, as might be expected from the analysis of individual criterion-referenced variables none of the differences were statistically significant, probably because of the large standard deviations which are a feature of these data.

In summary, there is no support for Prediction 1 because there is no evidence of superior rates of progress in the group receiving conductive education.

6.8.4   Variability in Criterion-Referenced Data (Prediction 2)

Figures 6.1–6.47 report standard deviations for the Birmingham and Manchester groups on 47 criterion-referenced variables at Time 1, Time 2 and Time 3 where data are available. Variance at Time 3 was compared to variance at Time 1 for the Birmingham and Manchester groups separately, but no interpretable pattern of results emerged.

For the Birmingham group, variance decreased significantly on two preverbal communication variables (Figures 6.17, 6.19) and three fine-motor variables (Figures 6.23, 6.28, 6.29), variance increased significantly on two cognitive variables (Figures 6.7, 6.10), three motor variables (Figures 6.3, 6.26, 6.35) and two physical variables (Figures 6.38, 6.40), but variance did not change significantly on the other 35 variables.

For the Manchester group, variance decreased significantly on two preverbal communication variables (Figures 6.17, 6.20), variance increased significantly on one cognitive variable (Figure 6.8), four motor variables (Figures 6.24, 6.26, 6.35, 6.36) and one physical variable (Figure 6.40), but variance did not change significantly on the other 39 variables.

Although there was less variability among the Birmingham children in their programme compared to the Manchester children (Section 6.7.3.3), there is no support for Prediction 2 that variance among children receiving conductive education should decrease more than variance in a group receiving United Kingdom special education.

6.8.5 Norm-Referenced Data

Figures 6.55–6.74 give the results of 20 norm-referenced variables in the order described in Section 6.2. All the figures have a similar form. In brackets at the top is the number of the Section which describes the variable. The data are plotted and 'age' on the ordinate refers to 'developmental age', 'age equivalent' or 'mental age' depending on the test. There is a table giving the size (N), mean, and standard deviation (SD) of the Birmingham and Manchester groups at Time 1, Time 2 and Time 3. At the bottom is a table summarising the results of a two-way univariate analysis of variance and t tests are reported comparing Time 1 with Time 2 and Time 2 with Time 3 performance.

6.8.5.1 Group Differences

The groups do not differ on any variable.

6.8.5.2 Time Differences

All variables yielded a significant Time effect except for the two measures of Intelligence Quotient (Figure 6.56, Figure 6.68) and Articulation (Figure 6.69). While the measures of Intelligence Quotient should not change because they are ratios of chronological age, it could have been expected that the Articulation variable would have shown improvement over time.

An examination of the plots of all the data and the results of the t tests at the bottom of the figures indicate that some variables show greater improvement between Time 1 and Time 2 than between Time 2 and Time 3. There is, however, no evidence for 'ceiling effects' because Time 3 means are well below the top of the scales.

The period between Time 1 and Time 3 assessments was 24 months. If the groups developed at the same rate as non-disabled children, their 'developmental age' at Time 3 should equal Time 1 plus 24 months. Figures 6.55–6.74 show, however, that 'developmental age' at Time 3 was less than Time 1 plus 24 months in all but two instances. In other words, the chidren tended to develop at a slower rate than predicted by age-norms.

The important conclusion, however, is that all but one of the variables which could be expected to change over time, were responsive to changes in the children.

6.8.5.3 Differential Change Over Time

Only two variables showed a significant Group × Time interaction. On Articulation (Figure 6.69) the Manchester group tended to improve while the Birmingham group tended to deteriorate. On Play (Figure 6.73) the groups showed a different pattern of improvement with the Manchester group improving more than the Birmingham group between Time 1 and Time 2, while the Birmingham group improved more than the Manchester group between Time 2 and Time 3. However, the importance of these isolated results is negligible given that the groups did not differ in their progress on the other 18 norm-referenced variables.

6.8.5.4   Discussion (Prediction 3)

There is no evidence to support Prediction 3 (Section 3.7) that conductive education should result in better progress on norm-referenced tests of function than United Kingdom special education. Conductive education failed, at least in the short term, to achieve goals implied by some definitions of orthofunction.

6.8.6   Conclusions

Prediction 1. While children receiving conductive education made progress on a wide range of functional and physical measures, they failed to achieve better rates of progress than children enrolled in United Kingdom special education.

Prediction 2. Over a wide range of functional and physical measures, variance among children receiving conductive education did not decrease more than variance among children receiving United Kingdom special education.

Prediction 3. Conductive education did not result in greater progress on norm-referenced tests of function than United Kingdom special education. Conductive education failed to achieve goals implied by some definitions of orthofunction.

6.9   INDIVIDUAL DIFFERENCES

6.9.1   Introduction

All children in the Birmingham group were specifically selected to benefit from conductive education, and given the high expectations generated by conductive education, the predictions outlined in Section 3.7, and the collateral data which, on balance, favoured conductive education, the group as a whole was expected to progress better than a matched group in Manchester which was receiving United Kingdom special education. This was not found. On the contrary, the only differences between the groups in their progress was in favour of the Manchester group.

While Objective 3 of the evaluation has been formally met in the analyses reported in Section 6.8, further attempts to seek out possible benefits of conductive education were undertaken. It can be expected that children will differ in their progress; the issue investigated was therefore whether it is possible to predict which children will benefit most.

6.9.2 Relationship Between State at Time 1 and Progress over the Time 1 to Time 3 Period

The following 39 Time 1 functional and physical variables were selected (section numbers describing the variables are in brackets): Academic (6.2.2.1), Communication (6.2.2.2), Physical (6.2.2.3), Social (6.2.2.4), Self-Help (6.2.2.5), General Cognition (6.2.3.7), Motor Control 1 (6.2.5.1.1), Motor Control 2 (6.2.5.1.2), Motor Control 3 (6.2.5.2.1), Receptive Non-Verbal (6.2.5.2.2), Expressive Non-Verbal (6.2.5.2.3), Receptive Verbal (6.2.5.2.4), Articulation (6.2.5.3), Expressive Verbal (6.2.5.4), Fine-Motor Independence (6.2.6.1), Object Transfer 1 (6.2.6.2), Object Transfer 2 (6.2.6.3), Manipulation (6.2.6.4), Two-Hand Coordination (6.2.6.5), Pen Placement (62.6.6), Drawing (6.2.6.7), Postural Independence (6.2.7.1), Position Changing Independence (6.2.7.2), Locomotion Independence (6.2.7.6), Position Changing (6.2.7.7), Crawling (6.2.7.8), Walking (6.2.7.9), Preferred Locomotion (6.2.7.10), Hip Mobility (6.2.8.1), Hamstring Extensibility (6.2.8.2), Height (6.2.8.3), Weight (6.2.8.4), Neurological Assessment (6.2.8.5), Gross-Motor (6.2.9.1), Interpersonal (6.2.9.2), Play (6.2.9.3), Activities of Daily Living (6.2.9.4), Attention and Control (6.2.9.5), Behaviour Problems (6.2.10).

The following seven Factor scores were calculated at Time 1 and Time giving global measures which summarise each child's functioning (Section 6.6.4): Factor 1 (Gross-Motor), Factor 2 (Expressive Language), Factor 4 (Cognitive and Social), Factor 5 (Independence and Motor), Factor 6 Physical and Gross-Motor), Factor 8 (Behaviour Problems), Factor 10 (Independence and Social). For each Factor, the difference between Time 3 and Time 1 gives a global measure of progress encompassing a range of inter-correlated variables.

6.9.2.1 Birmingham Group

Correlations between 39 Time 1 variables and the seven global measures of progress are based on 17 children who had complete assessment records. Only 27 of the 273 correlation coefficients were significant and these are given in Table 6.27.

Most of the significant correlations were found with Factor 1 (Gross-Motor). The higher the children's scores on a range of variables concerning motor function (Physical, Self-Help, Motor Control 1, Motor Control 2, Fine-Motor Independence, Object Transfer 1, Object Transfer 2, Manipulation, Postural Independence, Position Changing, Independence, Locomotion Independence, Position Changing, Preferred Locomotion, Gross-Motor, Activities of Daily Living), and on a range of scores concerning social behaviour (Social, Interpersonal, Play), the greater the progress on a pool of gross-motor variables making up Factor 1. In addition, the higher the children's general cognitive ability (General Cognition) the greater the progress on gross-motor variables, as might be predicted (Section 6.2.3). Also, the better the Neurological Assessment the greater the progress on gross-motor variables, which provides some validation for Bleck's (1975) prognostic procedure (Section 6.2.8.5). Overall, these results indicate that among children suitable for conductive education, those with milder motor problems, better social behaviour, higher general cognitive abilities and better neurological status will improve more in gross-motor functioning than more severely affected children.

The correlations between Self-Help at Time 1, Motor Control 1 at Time 1 and improvement on Factor 6 (Physical and Gross-Motor) are related to the correlations with improvement on Factor 1 (Gross-Motor) discussed above. The other scattered significant correlations in Table 6.27 are generally uninterpretable (eg., negative correlation between Height at Time 1 and improvement on Factor 2 (Expressive Language), positive correlation between Weight at Time 1 and improvement on Factor 10 (Independence and Social)).

Overall, it is striking that while performance at Time 1 on many variables is related to improvement in Gross-Motor functioning, performance at Time 1 is scarcely related to improvement on any of the other Factors relevant to expressive language, social behaviour, cognitive ability and independence in activities of daily living. Given that all the children were selected to benefit from conductive education, perhaps the general absence of correlations is a partial vindication of conductive education; ie., except for gross-motor functioning, the children's progress is not related to their intial state.

6.9.2.2   Manchester Group

Correlations between 39 Time 1 variables and the seven global measures of progress are based on 15 children who had complete assessment records. Fifty of the 273 correlation coefficients were significant and these are given in Table 6.28.

The Manchester group is 'incomplete' in the sense that only a small subset of children enrolled in schools in Manchester were selected for the study (Section 6.5). The pattern of correlations in Table 6.28 concerns only the relationship between initial state and progress among children suitable for conductive education but enrolled in United Kingdom special education, and a different pattern might well have occurred if all children in the Manchester schools had been included. Nonetheless, it is worthwhile considering the pattern of correlations as a contrast to the pattern found for the Birmingham group (Table 6.27).

The Time 1 variables which yielded significant correlations with progress on Factor scores are almost exclusively motor and physical variables, and these variables correlate with improvement on Factors covering a wide range of domains including motor functioning, expressive language, cognition, social behaviour and independence in activities of daily living. In other words, the Manchester children's progress in many domains is related to their initial motor and physical state. This contrasts with the pattern found for similar children enrolled in conductive education (Section 6.9.2.1), which indicated that except for progress in gross-motor functioning, progress is generally independent of initial state.

6.9.3 Discussion

The fact that similar children enrolled in United Kingdom special education and conductive education yield different patterns of correlations between initial state and subsequent progress, indicates that the general absence of correlations in the group receiving conductive education is, indeed, a function of the conductive education programme. This provides evidence that conductive education is, at least partially, achieving an aim of promoting the development of selected children regardless of their initial state. Ironically however, the aim is not met in regard to the promotion of motor functioning which seems to depend on a range of initial abilities.

These findings do not mean, however, that all children in conductive education made the same amount of progress (see also Section 7.6 and Section 7.7). On the contrary, children differed widely in their progress on the Factor scores and also with respect to the attainment of orthofunctional goals reviewed in the first part of Section 5.3. Two children who made the greatest progress on the factor scores and two children who made the least progress on the factor scores are chosen to illustrate this point.

One child with a moderate 'severity rating' from the conductors, who ranked generally high on initial research assessments of general cognition, language, motor functioning, social behaviour and independence in activities of daily living, made generally good progress on the Factor scores and was discharged into a mainstream school. It can be argued that conductive education was a 'success' for this child.

Another child with a moderate 'severity rating' from the conductors but who ranked generally low on initial research assessments, made generally good progress on the Factor scores but was not discharged from the Institute. It would be difficult to argue unequivocally that conductive education was a 'success' for this child.

On the other hand, there was a child with a severe 'severity rating' from the conductors, virtually no expressive language and a low ranking on initial research assessments except for a superior general cognitive ability, who made poor progress on all the Factor scores and was not discharged from the Institute. There was another child with a severe 'severity rating', good expressive language but a moderate to low ranking on all other initial research assessments, who also made poor progress on the Factor scores and was discharged into a special school. While the needs of these two children were great, it can be argued that conductive education failed to meet them.

Children in the Manchester group also varied in their progress on the Factor scores. However, a definition of the objectives of the Manchester programmes was not a requirement of the present evaluation and all children enrolled in them were not studied. The objectives for all children in the Manchester programmes may not include orthofunctional-type goals or discharge into mainstream schools, hence it is not possible to discuss the range of 'successes' and 'failures' that may exist.

6.10   CONCLUSIONS

i.   A group of children enrolled in programmes of United Kingdom special education in Greater Manchester were identified who matched a group enrolled in the Birmingham Institute on data ranging over a number of conductor assessments and research assessments, and over direct and indirect measures of functional abilities in different domains.

ii.   Comparing the progress of all children enrolled in the Birmingham Institute to that of a small subset of children enrolled in schools in Greater Manchester, provides a test of the efficacy of conductive education against a standard provided by United Kingdom special education, but does not provide a general test of the efficacy of United Kingdom special education because results in Manchester are only relevant to children who are acceptable for conductive education.

iii.   Most of the previously published tests used in the assessment battery report acceptable data on reliability and concurrent validity, while data on some of the newly developed tests indicate high test-retest reliability and high inter-rater reliability.

iv.   At the first assessment, performance on all parts of the assessment battery correlated poorly with chronological age, hence, chronological age was not a covariate of raw test data. In addition, chronological age was not considered to be a covariate of change in function over the Time 1 to Time 3 period.

v.   High correlations at the first assessment between variables within the domains of general cognition, receptive and expressive language, fine-motor functioning, gross-motor functioning, social behaviour, and independence in activities of daily living gave strong evidence of concurrent validity of the individual tests.

vi.   A Principal-Components Analysis of data from 41 functional and physical variables at the first assessment identified seven factors with interpretable patterns of association between variables. This provided a way of calculating seven global Factor scores which summarised each child's functioning at the first and last assessment.

vii. The two groups were closely matched on educational experiences prior to the first assessment, social class, and frequency of the following: mother's ethnic grouping, 'one-parent' and 'two-parent' families, family size.

viii. There was an indication that while the Birmingham mothers appreciated the time and effort expended by staff of the Institute on the children, they did not register an additional 'pay off' in terms of development. Also, there was a fall over time in 'satisfaction with progress' among the Birmingham parents but not among the Manchester parents.

ix.   The groups did not differ and there was no major change over time in a range of 'out-of-school' factors which could possibly have affected the progress of the children.

x.   There was no major difference between the groups with respect to change in educational experiences during the period of the evaluation, with similar numbers of children being discharged into mainstream schools.

xi.   The Birmingham group had more days of education available in each 12 month period than the Manchester group, but percentage absenteeism was similar in the two groups over the period of the evaluation.

xii. Comparisons between the timetables followed by the two groups led to the following conclusions: while there was virtually no variability in the timetable followed by the Birmingham group, each child in the Manchester group had an individual timetable; the Birmingham timetable had a four-fold longer amount of time allocated to programmes of a clearly physical nature but half the time allocated to programmes of a clearly academic nature compared to the Manchester timetable; the Manchester children were virtually free of exposure to conductive education.

xiii. According to staff, conductive education focused significantly more on functions assessed by the research team under the headings of 'fine-motor functioning', 'gross-motor functioning' and 'self-help behaviour' than programmes in Manchester.

xiv. Longitudinal comparisons between the groups on data from 47 criterion-referenced variables led to the following conclusions:

Nearly all the functional variables were responsive to changes in the children.

Children receiving conductive education made progress on a wide range of measures.

Contrary to Prediction 1 that children receiving conductive education would make better progress than children receiving United Kingdom special education, the only evidence of differences in the functional development of the groups was in favour of the group receiving Untied Kingdom special education.

A deterioration in the mobility of the hips in the group receiving conductive education, when no such deterioration was seen in the Manchester group, may reflect an inadequate consideration in conductive education of the orthopaedic problems of children with cerebral palsy.

xv. Longitudinal comparisons between the groups on seven Factor scores which pool the 47 criterion-referenced variables led to the following conclusions: all Factor scores were responsive to changes in the children; while children receiving conductive education made substantial progress on a wide range of measures, there was no support for Prediction 1 because there was no evidence of superior rates of progress compared to the Manchester group.

xvi. An investigation of change in variance within the Birmingham and Manchester groups found no support for Prediction 2 that variance among children receiving conductive education should decrease more than variance in a group receiving United Kingdom special education.

xvii. Longitudinal comparisons between the groups on data from 20 norm-referenced variables led to the following conclusions: all but one of the variables which would be expected to change over time, were responsive to changes in the children; there was no evidence to support Prediction 3 that conductive education should result in better progress on norm-referenced tests of function than United Kingdom special education. Hence, conductive education failed, at least in the short-term, to achieve goals implied by some definitions of orthofunction.

xviii. Given the following advantages for the group receiving conductive education compared to the group receiving United Kingdom special education—greater specificity in the selection and grouping of children, longer exposure to the programme in each year, greater exposure to programmes of a clearly physical nature and staff's higher rating to the 'relevance' of the fine-motor, gross-motor and self-help research assessments—the lack of any evidence of superior rates of progress in the group receiving conductive education can only be interpreted as failure of conductive education in Birmingham to fulfil the high expectations which have come to be associated with this system.

xix. An examination of individual differences in progress among children receiving conductive education suggests that conductive education is, at least partially, achieving an aim of promoting the development of selected children regardless of the initial state of these children, although perhaps ironically, the aim is not met in regard to the promotion of motor functioning because the amount of progress made by children in this regard is related to a range of initial abilities.

xx. Children receiving conductive education differed widely in their progress and while it can be argued that conductive education was a 'success' for some children, equally it can be argued that it was a 'failure' for other children.

xxi. The evaluation does not provide a general test of the efficacy of United Kingdom special education and although the results cannot be taken as a vindication of methods employed, until it can be demonstrated that conductive education meets the expectations of its protagonists, the following conclusions are appropriate: staff involved with United Kingdom special education should be circumspect in their view of conductive education and should not feel compelled to adopt the methods which are advocated; parents of children with cerebral palsy should regard with caution the promises made on behalf of conductive education and they should not feel they are failing if they do not secure conductive education for their child.

Table 6.1 **A comparison between Intake 1 and Intake 2 of the Birmingham Institute at the time of the first research assessment centred on 1 January 1989.**

Variable		Intake 1	Intake 2	Comparison
Age at 1.1.89	Mean	61.0	61.0	
	SD	6.8	8.5	
Period since first involved in education*	Mean	44.5	40.9	t(16)0.68, ns
	SD	10.0	12.6	
Developmental Profile II†				
Self-help scale	Mean	−25.1	−26.5	t(15)0.19, ns
	SD	9.6	18.8	
Social scale	Mean	−2.2	−7.5	t(15)0.89, ns
	SD	8.2	15.6	
Communication scale	Mean	−11.8	−6.0	t(15)0.71, ns
	SD	14.4	18.9	
Gross-motor independence	Median	32	32	
	Range	28–50	26–52	
Fine-motor function‡				
Preferred-hand	Mean	0.25	0.22	t(16)0.44, ns
	SD	0.13	0.15	
Non preferred-hand	Mean	0.21	0.19	t(16)0.28, ns
	SD	0.13	0.17	

* months
† months differential
‡ balls/sec

Table 6.2 **Comparison between children in the Birmingham group (Time 1 assessment of Intake 1 and Intake 2) and children in the Manchester group (screening assessments).**

Variable		Birmingham	Manchester	Comparison
Age in months*	Mean	61.0	55.4	t = 2.16,
	SD	7.3	8.5	df = 36,
				p<.05
Conductors' diagnosis (Quad. Di. Athet. At.)	Frequency	11:3:2:2	9:5:4:2	
Conductors' severity rating (Sev. Mod. Mild)	Frequency	10:4:4	6:6:8	x^2 = 2.64, df = 2, ns
Developmental Profile II†				
Self-help scale	Mean	−25.8	−25.0	t = 0.15,
	SD	14.2	17.2	df = 35, ns
Social scale	Mean	−4.7	−15.1	t = 2.17,
	SD	12.1	16.3	df = 35,
				p<.05
Communication scale	Mean	−9.1	−11.4	t = 0.38,
	SD	16.4	20.6	df = 35, ns
Gross-motor independence	Median	32.0	36.0	U = 171,
	Range	26–52	21–52	n_1 = 18,
				n_2 = 20, ns
Fine-motor function‡				
Preferred-hand	Mean	0.23	0.23	
	SD	0.13	0.15	
Non preferred-hand	Mean	0.20	0.15	t = 1.15,
	SD	0.14	0.15	df = 35, ns

* Birmingham group 1 January 1989, Manchester group 1 January 1990.

† months differential (one Birmingham parent unavailable for interview).

‡ balls/sec

Table 6.3 Comparison between the child in the Birmingham group who was withdrawn from the evaluation (code 14) and the next eight lowest scoring children in the group (code 12, 20, 18, 4, 2, 9, 10, 16) on Time 1 assessment data.

Variable	Child								
	14	12	20	18	4	2	9	10	16
Developmental Profile†									
Mean	−49.2	−29.4	−25.8	−24.8	−24.0	−23.8	−23.4	−23.4	−19.2
SD	11.1	19.0	17.1	15.8	13.6	15.3	16.1	15.5	14.7
Number of Direct Assessments With Score Greater than Zero*	5	14	15	14	12	12	14	14	12

† months differential
* maximum 15

Table 6.4 Comparison between three children in the Manchester group (code 31, 38, 43) like the withdrawn Birmingham child (code 14) and the next six lowest scoring children in the group (code 41, 34, 39, 49, 37, 40) on Time 1 assessment data.

Variable	Child								
	31	38	43	41	34	39	49	37	40
Developmental Profile†									
Mean	−45.8	−47.4	−35.0	−48.0	−33.2	−30.8	−29.2	−24.6	−19.8
SD	5.1	12.1	5.8	9.5	13.9	17.2	6.9	13.5	11.5
Number of Direct Assessments with Score Greater than Zero*	4	7	5	13	13	10	4	15	14

† months differential
* maximum 15

Table 6.5 Test-retest reliability: relationship between raw scores obtained on Developmental Profile II at Time 1 and an interim assessment, for children in Intakes 1 and 2 of the Birmingham group (N = 16).

Scale		Time 1	Interim Assessment	t	r
Academic	M	16.8	20.2	4.04	0.65
	SD	4.1	3.9	p<.01	
Communication	M	21.9	25.4	4.82	0.90
	SD	5.6	6.5	p<.001	
Physical	M	8.8	10.6	2.70	0.81
	SD	4.2	4.4	p<.02	
Social	M	22.7	24.2	2.30	0.54
	SD	2.2	3.0	p<.05	
Self-Help	M	15.3	19.4	4.44	0.84
	SD	5.3	6.7	p<0.001	

Table 6.6 Test-retest reliability: relationship between raw scores obtained on the Fine-Motor Assessment at Time 1 and an interim assessment, for children in Intakes 1 and 2 of the Birmingham group (N = 17).

Scale		Time 1	Interim Assessment	t	r
Independence	M	27.6	29.8	1.23	0.54
	SD	8.7	4.2	ns	
Object Transfer 1	M	0.17	0.18	1.20	0.94
	SD	0.12	0.11	ns	
Object Transfer 2	M	0.23	0.25	1.31	0.89
	SD	0.12	0.14	ns	
Manipulation	M	1.00	1.38	3.70	0.78
	SD	0.66	0.60	p<.01	
Two-Hand Coordination	M	0.03	0.04	2.84	0.68
	SD	0.01	0.01	p<.05	
Pen Placement	M	−25.8	−4.0	1.27	0.88
	SD	74.1	3.6	ns	
Drawing	M	−27.9	−8.7	1.64	0.77
	SD	58.3	13.9	ns	

Table 6.7 Test-retest reliability: relationship between raw scores obtained on the Adaptive Behaviour scales at Time 1 and an interim assessment, for children in Intakes 1 and 2 of the Birmingham group (N = 17).

Scale		Time 1	Interim Assessment	t	r
Gross Motor	M	28.6	25.3	1.66	0.91
	SD	14.7	19.3	ns	
Interpersonal	M	19.4	16.1	2.65	0.75
	SD	6.1	7.7	p<.05	
Play	M	13.1	10.6	4.06	0.80
	SD	4.1	3.1	p<.01	
Activities of Daily Living	M	31.9	25.6	4.32	0.92
	SD	11.9	7.2	p<.01	
Attention and Control	M	23.5	27.4	4.09	0.75
	SD	5.9	5.1	p<.01	

Table 6.8 Inter-rater reliability: relationship between raw scores obtained by two judges who independently derived data from video-recordings of the Time 1 Fine-Motor assessment of Intakes 1 and 2 of the Birmingham group according to written criteria (N = 17).

Scale		Judge 1	Judge 2	r
Independence	M	27.6	26.1	0.92
	SD	8.7	9.2	
Object Transfer 1	M	0.17	0.17	1.00
	SD	0.12	0.12	
Object Transfer 2	M	0.23	0.23	1.00
	SD	0.12	0.12	
Manipulation	M	1.00	1.00	1.00
	SD	0.66	0.64	
Two-Hand Coordination	M	0.031	0.031	1.00
	SD	0.014	0.014	
Pen Placement	M	−25.8	−39.4	0.84
	SD	74.1	100.1	
Drawing	M	−27.9	−37.8	0.82
	SD	58.3	72.6	

Table 6.9 Inter-rater reliability: relationship between raw scores obtained by two judges who independently derived data from video recordings of the Time 1 Gross-Motor Assessment of five children in the Manchester group according to written criteria.

Scale		Judge 1	Judge 2	r
Postural Independence	M	16.8	17.0	0.98
	SD	3.3	3.4	
Position Change Independence	M	17.2	17.4	0.99
	SD	5.3	5.0	
Crawling Independence	M	3	3	1.00
	SD	0	0	
Walking Independence	M	2.0	2.0	1.00
	SD	1.0	1.0	
Preferred Locomotion Independence	M	2.0	2.0	1.00
	SD	1.0	1.0	
Position Changing	M	24.3	24.6	0.95
	SD	12.4	12.3	
Crawling	M	16.9	16.9	0.98
	SD	17.1	17.1	
Walking	M	16.3	16.2	0.97
	SD	13.7	13.7	
Preferred Locomotion	M	23.8	24.4	0.98
	SD	29.2	29.1	

Table 6.10   Correlations between 10 tests of receptive and expressive language, based on Time 1 raw score data from 35 children in the Birmingham and Manchester groups.

Test					Test					
	1	2	3	4	5	6	7	8	9	10
1. Developmental Profile II: Communication	1.00	0.44**	0.80**	0.73**	0.53**	0.81**	0.60**	0.47**	0.47**	0.85*
2. Receptive Non-Verbal		1.00	0.64*	0.35*	0.20	0.50**	0.23	0.41*	0.93**	0.35*
3. Expressive Non-Verbal			1.00	0.76**	0.44**	0.98**	0.50**	0.29	0.62**	0.82*
4. Motor Control 1				1.00	0.77**	0.79**	0.78**	0.22	0.35*	0.84*
5. Motor Control 2					1.00	0.45**	0.59**	0.22	0.19	0.63*
6. Motor Control 3						1.00	0.52**	0.20	0.49**	0.85*
7. Articulation							1.00	0.42*	0.31	0.75*
8. Pictorial Test of Intelligence: General Cognition								1.00	0.58**	0.29
9. Receptive Verbal									1.00	0.40*
10. Expressive Verbal										1.00

* p<.05 two tailed
** p<.01 two tailed

151

Table 6.11 **Correlations between eight tests concerned with fine-motor functioning, based on Time 1 raw score data from 35 children in the Birmingham and Manchester groups.**

Test				Test				
	1	2	3	4	5	6	7	8
1. Developmental Profile II: Physical	1.00	0.61**	0.71**	0.59**	0.65**	0.48**	0.30**	0.38**
2. Independence		1.00	0.70**	0.60*	0.70**	0.42**	0.70**	0.83**
3. Object Transfer 1			1.00	0.70**	0.64**	0.58**	0.40*	0.49**
4. Object Transfer 2				1.00	0.62**	0.50**	0.36*	0.43*
5. Manipulation					1.00	0.42*	0.38*	0.47**
6. Two-Hand Coordination						1.00	0.30	0.32
7. Pen Placement							1.00	0.87**
8. Drawing								1.00

* p<.05 two tailed
** p<.01 two tailed

Table 6.12 Correlations between 11 tests of gross-motor functioning, based on Time 1 raw score data from 35 children in the Birmingham and Manchester groups.

Test						Test					
	1	2	3	4	5	6	7	8	9	10	11
1. Developmental Profile II: Physical	1.00	0.79**	0.65**	0.72**	0.59**	0.53**	0.31	0.77**	0.54**	0.55**	0.70**
2. Adaptive Behaviour: Gross-Motor		1.00	0.74**	0.85**	0.75**	0.69**	0.31	0.76**	0.55**	0.66**	0.64**
3. Postural Independence			1.00	0.91**	0.64**	0.54**	0.40*	0.72**	0.26	0.52**	0.41*
4. Position Changing Independence				1.00	0.73**	0.58**	0.45**	0.84**	0.35*	0.56**	0.50**
5. Crawling Independence					1.00	0.59**	0.26	0.75**	0.63**	0.73**	0.65**
6. Walking Independence						1.00	0.12	0.61**	0.47**	0.79**	0.34*
7. Preferred Locomotion Independence							1.00	0.42*	0.18	0.17	0.33
8. Position Changing								1.00	0.57**	0.64**	0.69**
9. Crawling									1.00	0.58**	0.82**
10. Walking										1.00	0.60**
11. Preferred Locomotion											1.00

* p<.05 two tailed
** p<.01 two tailed

Table 6.13 **Correlations between three tests of social functioning, based on Time 1 raw score data from 35 children in the Birmingham and Manchester groups.**

Test		Test	
	1	2	3
1. Developmental Profile II: Social	1.00	0.56**	0.56**
2. Adaptive Behaviour: Interpersonal Relationship		1.00	0.86**
3. Adaptive Behaviour: Play			1.00

** p<.01 two tailed

Table 6.14 **Ten factors identified in a principal-components analysis of 41 functional and physical variables (Appendix 6.4) at Time 1.**

Factor	Eigenvalue	Per cent of Variance	Cumulative Per cent
1	15.70	38.3	38.3
2	4.87	11.9	50.2
3	3.07	7.5	57.7
4	2.82	6.9	64.5
5	1.86	4.5	69.1
6	1.75	4.3	73.4
7	1.61	3.9	77.3
8	1.33	3.2	80.5
9	1.15	2.8	83.3
10	1.05	2.6	85.9

Table 6.15 Seven factors identified in a principal-components analysis of 41 functional and physical variables (Appendix 6.4) at Time 1, which show interpretable patterns of association between variables, after varimax rotation and Kaiser normalisation.

Factor	Title	Variables	Loadings
1	'Gross-Motor'	Gross-Motor: Walking	0.863
		Gross-Motor: Crawling	0.834
		Gross-Motor: Crawling Independence	0.772
		Gross-Motor: Preferred Locomotion	0.744
		Gross-Motor: Walking Independence	0.743
		Gross-Motor: Position Changing	0.697
		Adaptive Behaviour: Gross-Motor	0.664
		Developmental Profile II: Physical	0.544
		Gross-Motor: Position Changing Independence	0.514
2	'Expressive Language'	Language: Expressive Verbal	0.911
		Language: Motor Control 3	0.872
		Developmental Profile II: Communication	0.846
		Language: Motor Control 1	0.826
		Language: Expressive Non-Verbal	0.824
		Language: Articulation	0.739
		Language: Motor Control 2	0.513
4	'Cognitive and Social'	Adaptive Behaviour: Play	0.891
		Pictorial Test of Intelligence: General Cognition	0.854
		Adaptive Behaviour: Interpersonal	0.792
		Adaptive Behaviour: Attention and Control	0.683
		Developmental Profile II: Academic	0.571
		Developmental Profile II: Social	0.567
5	'Independence and Motor'	Fine-Motor: Object Transfer 2	0.724
		Fine-Motor: Manipulation	0.630
		Fine-Motor: Object Transfer 1	0.604
		Language: Motor Control 2	0.603
		Physical: Neurology	0.564
		Adaptive Behaviour: Activities of Daily Living	0.485
		Fine-Motor: Independence	0.444
		Adaptive Behaviour: Gross Motor	0.443

Table 6.15—continued

Factor	Title	Variables	Loadings
6	'Physical and Gross-Motor'	Physical: Hamstring Extensibility	0.792
		Physical: Hip Mobility	0.645
		Gross-Motor: Postural Independence	0.569
		Gross-Motor: Position Changing Independence	0.568
		Gross-Motor: Position Changing	0.420
		Adaptive Behaviour: Gross	0.412
		Gross-Motor: Walking Independence	0.377
8	'Behaviour Problems'	Behaviour Problems	0.914
10	'Independence and Social'	Developmental Profile II: Self-Help	0.428
		Developmental Profile II: Academic	0.362
		Developmental Profile II: Social	0.318

Table 6.16 **Comparison between the Birmingham and Manchester group on educational experiences of the children before Time 1 assessments. Data are in months.**

Variable		Birmingham	Manchester	Comparison
Age at first 'educational' intervention	M	17.8	14.6	t = 0.90, df = 34, ns
	SD	11.6	9.1	
Period between first intervention and Time 1 assessments	M	42.5	40.4	t = 0.59, df = 34, ns
	SD	10.8	11.3	

Table 6.17 Comparison between the Birmingham and Manchester groups on frequency of social class of the families.

Social Class	Birmingham	Manchester
I and II	8	4
IIIM and IIIN	4	6
IV and V	2	3
Unemployed	5	4

Table 6.18 Comparison between the Birmingham and Manchester groups on the frequency of various factors relating to the families at Time 1.

		Birmingham	Manchester
Mother's ethnic group	White	17	17
	Non-white	2	0
Family	Two-parent	16	17
	Single-parent	3	0
Number of children	One	3	3
in the family	Two	9	6
	More than two	7	8

Table 6.19 Comparison between the Birmingham and Manchester groups on mothers' psychological well-being, mothers' feeling about her life as a whole, mothers' feeling about the help received by her child and mothers' feeling about the progress being made by her child at Time 1, Time 2 and Time 3.

		Time 1		Time 2		Time 3	
		B'ham	Manchester	B'ham	Manchester	B'ham	Manchester
Mothers' psychological well-being	N	19	17	18	16	19	17
	Mean	20.1	19.4	19.2	19.0	18.9	18.8
	SD	4.0	4.5	5.7	3.4	6.2	4.5
Mothers' feeling about life as a whole	N	19	16	18	15	18	17
	Mean	6.4	5.9	6.5	6.7	7.1	6.7
	SD	2.0	2.4	2.1	1.5	1.5	1.3
Mothers' feeling about help received by her child	N	19	17	18	15	19	17
	Mean	8.4	6.6	8.6	6.7	8.0	6.4
	SD	1.0	2.1	0.8	1.9	1.3	2.3
Mothers' feeling about progress made by child	N	19	17	18	15	19	17
	Mean	6.9	6.4	7.2	6.4	7.2	6.4
	SD	1.7	2.2	1.5	1.9	1.5	2.0

Table 6.20 Comparison between the Birmingham and Manchester groups on the parent's satisfaction with overall progress made by their children: number of parents in four categories of satisfaction, in the Time 1—Time 2 and Time 2—Time 3 period.

Category of Satisfaction	Time 1—Time 2 Birmingham	Manchester	Time 2—Time 3 Birmingham	Manchester
Very Satisfied	16	10	6	10
Satisfied	3	2	9	3
Mixed	0	2	4	4
Not Satisfied	0	3	0	0

Table 6.21 Number of times parents in the Birmingham (N = 19) and Manchester (N = 17) groups reported input under four categories (1. family input, 2. input from educational and paramedical professionals, 3. input from medical professionals, 4. other input) having helpful, hindering and uncertain effects on seven areas of function assessed by the research team during the period between Time 1 and Time 2 assessments.

Area of Function	Effect	Input Category 1		2		3		4		Total	
		B'ham	Man	B'ham	Man	B'ham	Man	B'ham	Man	B'ham	Man
Cognition	Help	44	35	1	0	0	0	0	1	45	36
	Hinder	1	0	0	0	2	0	4	1	7	1
	Uncertain	0	0	1	0	0	0	0	0	1	0
Communication	Help	34	17	0	1	0	0	1	0	35	18
	Hinder	0	0	0	0	0	0	3	2	3	2
	Uncertain	0	0	0	0	1	0	0	0	1	0
Fine-Motor	Help	20	25	1	1	0	0	0	1	21	27
	Hinder	0	0	0	0	0	1	1	1	1	2
	Uncertain	0	0	0	0	0	0	0	0	0	0
Gross-Motor	Help	34	34	4	1	1	0	5	1	44	36
	Hinder	2	0	1	1	4	2	5	1	12	4
	Uncertain	0	1	1	0	3	0	0	0	4	1
Personal	Help	20	15	0	0	0	0	2	0	22	15
	Hinder	0	1	0	0	0	0	9	17	9	18
	Uncertain	0	0	0	0	0	0	1	1	1	1

Table 6.21—continued

| Area of Function | Effect | Input Category | | | | | | | | | |
| | | 1 | | 2 | | 3 | | 4 | | Total | |
		B'ham	Man	B'ham	Man	B'ham	Man	B'ham	Man	B'ham	Man
Interpersonal	Help	27	24	0	0	0	0	6	8	33	32
	Hinder	0	0	0	0	2	0	4	2	6	2
	Uncertain	0	0	0	0	0	0	0	0	0	0
Self-Help	Help	27	29	1	1	0	0	2	0	30	30
	Hinder	0	0	2	0	0	0	1	1	3	1
	Uncertain	0	0	0	0	0	0	0	0	0	0
Total	Help	206	179	7	4	1	0	16	11	230	194
	Hinder	3	1	3	1	8	3	27	25	41	30
	Uncertain	0	1	2	0	4	0	1	1	7	2

Table 6.22 Number of times parents in the Birmingham (N = 19) and Manchester (N = 17) groups reported input under four categories (1. family input, 2. input from educational and paramedical professionals, 3. input from medical professionals, 4. other input) having helpful, hindering and uncertain effects on seven areas of function assessed by the research team during the period between Time 2 and Time 3 assessments.

Area of Function	Effect	Input Category									
		1		2		3		4		Total	
		B'ham	Man	B'ham	Man	B'ham	Man	B'ham	Man	B'ham	Man
Cognition	Help	56	36	0	0	0	0	1	1	57	37
	Hinder	0	0	0	0	0	0	3	1	3	1
	Uncertain	0	0	0	1	0	0	0	0	1	0
Communication	Help	23	16	0	0	0	0	1	3	24	19
	Hinder	0	0	0	0	1	0	2	1	2	2
	Uncertain	0	0	0	0	0	0	0	0	0	0
Fine-Motor	Help	29	29	0	0	0	0	0	1	29	30
	Hinder	0	0	0	0	0	0	1	0	1	0
	Uncertain	0	0	0	0	0	0	0	0	0	0
Gross-Motor	Help	43	35	3	7	4	1	5	1	56	43
	Hinder	0	0	1	1	1	0	7	2	8	4
	Uncertain	0	0	0	0	1	1	0	0	0	1
Personal	Help	15	11	0	0	0	0	3	4	18	15
	Hinder	0	2	0	0	2	0	11	5	11	9
	Uncertain	0	0	0	0	0	0	0	0	0	0

Table 6.22—continued

| Area of Function | Effect | Input Category | | | | | | | | Total | |
| | | 1 | | 2 | | 3 | | 4 | | | |
		B'ham	Man	B'ham	Man	B'ham	Man	B'ham	Man	B'ham	Man
Interpersonal	Help	30	19	0	0	0	0	8	9	38	28
	Hinder	0	0	0	0	0	0	0	2	0	2
	Uncertain	0	0	0	0	0	0	0	0	0	0
Self-Help	Help	28	23	0	0	0	0	0	0	28	23
	Hinder	0	0	0	0	0	0	0	0	0	0
	Uncertain	0	0	0	0	0	0	0	0	0	0
Total	Help	224	169	7	3	1	4	18	19	250	195
	Hinder	0	2	1	1	0	4	24	11	25	18
	Uncertain	0	0	1	0	0	1	0	0	1	1

Table 6.23 Comparison between the Birmingham and Manchester groups on the incidence of family input reported by parents as 'helpful' to areas of function assessed by the research team over the Time 1—Time 2 and Time 2—Time 3 periods.

Area of Function		Time 1—Time 2		Time 2—Time 3	
		Birmingham	Manchester	Birmingham	Manchester
Cognition	M	2.26	2.06	2.95	2.12
	SD	0.73	0.97	0.97	0.78
Communication	M	1.84	1.00	1.21	0.94
	SD	1.01	0.50	0.79	0.83
Fine-Motor	M	1.05	1.47	1.47	1.71
	SD	0.52	0.62	0.51	1.05
Gross-Motor	M	1.79	2.00	2.26	2.06
	SD	1.40	1.17	1.19	1.25
Personal	M	1.05	0.88	0.84	0.65
	SD	0.91	0.70	0.96	0.79
Interpersonal	M	1.42	2.06	1.58	1.12
	SD	1.02	0.75	0.96	0.60
Self-Help	M	1.42	1.06	1.47	1.35
	SD	1.17	0.56	0.70	0.61
All Areas	M	10.84	10.53	11.79	9.94
	SD	4.27	2.37	3.49	2.22

Table 6.24 Comparison between the Birmingham and Manchester groups on the number of children discharged into another programme of education in the Time 1—Time 2 and Time 2—Time 3 period.

	Time 1—Time 2		Time 2—Time 3		Total	
	B'ham	Man	B'ham	Man	B'ham	Man
Number of children discharged to mainstream schools	1	1	3	4	4	5
Number of children discharged to another special school	0	0	2	0	2	0

Table 6.25 Comparison between the Birmingham and Manchester groups on the number of half-days education available and the percentage of these half-days that children were absent in the Time 1—Time 2 and Time 2—Time 3 period.

| | | Time 1—Time 2 | | Time 2—Time 3 | |
		Birmingham	Manchester	Birmingham	Manchester
Number of half-days education available	M	393	378	381	375
	SD	3.5	11.5	6.9	1.9
Percentage of half-days available that children were absent	M	12.2	9.6	12.9	7.8
	SD	9.2	6.2	9.2	4.9

Table 6.26 Relevance of the research assessments to the programmes of education which were offered between the Time 1 and Time 2 assessments; mean and standard deviation of the sum of 'relevance' scores given to categories of function under each of seven headings for the Birmingham (N = 18) and Manchester (N = 17) groups.

Functional Heading		Birmingham	Manchester	Comparison
Mental Functioning	M	20.5	18.9	$t = 1.53$, df = 33, ns
	SD	2.6	3.6	
Communication	M	10.7	12.4	$t = 1.49$, df = 33, ns
	SD	3.4	3.5	
Fine-Motor Functioning	M	12.9	9.7	$t = 2.32$, df = 33, $p<.05$
	SD	3.5	4.8	
Gross-Motor Functioning	M	12.8	9.5	$5 = 3.87$, df = 33, $p<.001$
	SD	2.1	2.9	
Personal Behaviour	M	12.5	11.2	$t = 1.10$, df = 33, ns
	SD	3.2	3.6	
Interpersonal Behaviour	M	11.3	13.2	$t = 1.48$, df = 33, ns
	SD	4.1	3.7	
Self-Help Behaviour	M	22.9	19.1	$t = 2.63$, df = 33, $p<.05$
	SD	2.5	5.7	

Table 6.27 Relationship between state at Time 1 and progress over the Time 1 to Time 3 period: significant correlations between measures at Time 1 and the difference between Time 3 and Time 1 Factor scores for children in the Birmingham group.

Variable	Section Number	Factor (Time 3—Time 1)				
		1	2	6	8	10
Physical	6.2.2.3	+0.66**				
Social	6.2.2.4	+0.67**				
Self-Help	6.2.2.5	+0.78**		+0.55*		
General Cognition	6.2.3.7	+0.50*				
Motor Control 1	6.2.5.1.1	+0.64**		+0.50*		
Motor Control 2	6.2.5.1.2	+0.62**				
Articulation	6.2.5.3	+0.51*				
Expressive Verbal	6.2.5.4		−0.49*			
Fine-Motor Independence	6.2.6.1	+0.53*				
Object Transfer 1	6.2.6.2	+0.62**				
Object Transfer 2	6.2.6.3	+0.58*				
Manipulation	6.2.6.4	+0.73**				
Postural Independence	6.2.7.1	+0.50*				
Position Changing Independence	6.2.7.2	+0.62**				
Locomotion Independence	6.2.7.6	+0.76**				
Position Changing	6.2.7.7	+0.66**				
Preferred Locomotion	6.2.7.10	+0.81**				
Height	6.2.8.3		−0.55*			
Weight	6.2.8.4				+0.57*	+0.49*
Neurological Assessment	6.2.8.5	+0.57*				
Gross-Motor	6.2.9.1	+0.62**				
Interpersonal	6.2.9.2	+0.50*				
Play	6.2.9.3	+0.49*				
Activities of Daily Living	6.2.9.4	+0.78**				

* p<.05 ** p<.01, two=tailed.

Table 6.28 Relationship between state at Time 1 and progress over the Time 1 to Time 3 period significant correlations between measures at Time 1 and the difference between Time 3 and Time 1 Factor scores for children in the Manchester group.

Variable	Section Number	Factor (Time 3—Time 1)						
		1	2	4	5	6	8	10
Physical	6.2.2.3	+0.70**		+0.59*	+0.58*	+0.66**	+0.57*	+0.54*
Motor Control 1	6.2.5.1.1						+0.55*	
Motor Control 2	6.2.5.1.2	+0.61*		+0.66**	+0.63*		+0.77**	
Receptive Non-Verbal	6.2.5.2.2		−0.59*					
Receptive Verbal	6.2.5.2.4		−0.57*					
Object Transfer 1	6.2.6.2	+0.53*				+0.63*		
Object Transfer 2	6.2.6.3				+0.53*	+0.74**		
Manipulation	6.2.6.4	+0.59*					+0.61*	
Pen Placement	6.2.6.6		−0.56*					
Drawing	6.2.6.7		−0.54*					
Position Changing								
Independence	6.2.7.2	+0.61*						
Locomotion Independence	6.2.7.6	+0.55*						
Position Changing	6.2.7.7	+0.55*		+0.52*		+0.52*		
Crawling	6.2.7.8					+0.55*		+0.55*
Walking	6.2.7.9	+0.70**		+0.72**	+0.56*	+0.63*	+0.71**	+0.65**
Preferred Locomotion	6.2.7.10					+0.64**		+0.53*
Hamstring Extensibility	6.2.8.2	+0.74**			+0.64*		+0.58*	
Neurological Assessment	6.2.8.5		+0.54*					
Gross-Motor	6.2.9.1	+0.76**		+0.60*	+0.59*	+0.73**	+0.59*	+0.67**
Behaviour Problems	6.2.10	+0.57*				+0.58*		+0.60*

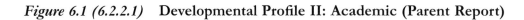

Figure 6.1 (6.2.2.1) Developmental Profile II: Academic (Parent Report)

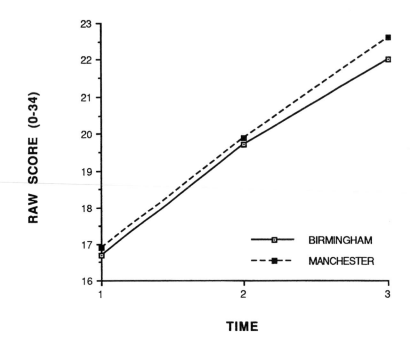

TIME

	TIME 1	TIME 2	TIME 3
BIRMINGHAM			
N	18	19	19
MEAN	16.7	19.7	22.0
SD	4.3	3.9	4.4
MANCHESTER			
N	17	17	17
MEAN	16.9	19.9	22.6
SD	5.0	4.9	5.9

SOURCE OF VARIATION	SUM OF SQUARES	df	Var. Est.	F	Sig.
GROUP	3.07	1,33	3.07	0.05	ns
TIME	528.55	2,66	264.27	69.70	<0.001
GROUP X TIME	1.24	2,66	0.62	0.16	ns

TIME 1 vs TIME 2, t=-6.69, df=34, p<0.001;
TIME 2 vs TIME 3, t=-6.45, df=35, p<0.001.

Figure 6.2 (6.2.2.2)   Developmental Profile II: Communication (Parent
Report)

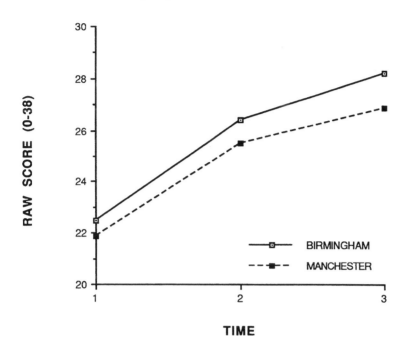

	TIME 1	TIME 2	TIME 3
BIRMINGHAM			
N	18	19	19
MEAN	22.5	26.4	28.2
SD	5.7	5.5	7.1
MANCHESTER			
N	17	17	17
MEAN	21.9	25.5	26.9
SD	6.9	7.4	7.0

SOURCE OF VARIATION	SUM OF SQUARES	df	Var. Est.	F	Sig.
GROUP	23.13	1,33	23.13	0.19	ns
TIME	527.27	2,66	263.63	58.01	<0.001
GROUP X TIME	1.44	2,66	0.72	0.16	ns

TIME 1 vs TIME 2, t=-8.43, df=34, p<0.001;
TIME 2 vs TIME 3, t=-3.43, df=35, p<0.05.

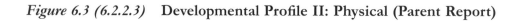

Figure 6.3 (6.2.2.3) Developmental Profile II: Physical (Parent Report)

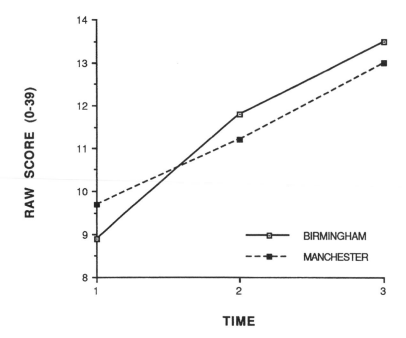

	TIME 1	TIME 2	TIME 3
BIRMINGHAM			
N	18	19	19
MEAN	8.9	11.8	13.5
SD	4.5	5.1	6.8
MANCHESTER			
N	17	17	17
MEAN	9.7	11.2	13.0
SD	4.3	5.0	6.4

SOURCE OF VARIATION	SUM OF SQUARES	df	Var. Est.	F	Sig.
GROUP	2.32	1,33	2.32	0.03	ns
TIME	294.47	2,66	147.24	31.50	<0.001
GROUP X TIME	14.70	2,66	7.35	1.57	ns

TIME 1 vs TIME 2, t=-5.13, df=34, p<0.001;
TIME 2 vs TIME 3, t=-3.65, df=35, p<0.05.

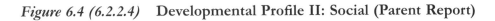

Figure 6.4 (6.2.2.4)   Developmental Profile II: Social (Parent Report)

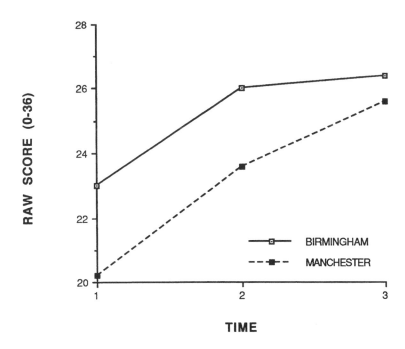

	TIME 1	TIME 2	TIME 3
BIRMINGHAM			
N	18	19	19
MEAN	23.0	26.0	26.4
SD	2.9	3.1	4.2
MANCHESTER			
N	17	17	17
MEAN	20.2	23.6	25.6
SD	4.9	4.7	4.5

SOURCE OF VARIATION	SUM OF SQUARES	df	Var. Est.	F	Sig.
GROUP	105.95	1,33	105.95	2.53	ns
TIME	363.40	2,66	181.70	38.09	<0.001
GROUP X TIME	21.34	2,66	10.67	2.24	ns

TIME 1 vs TIME 2, t=-6.41, df=34, p<0.001;
TIME 2 vs TIME 3, t=-2.39, df=35, p<0.05.

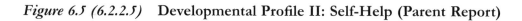

Figure 6.5 (6.2.2.5)   Developmental Profile II: Self-Help (Parent Report)

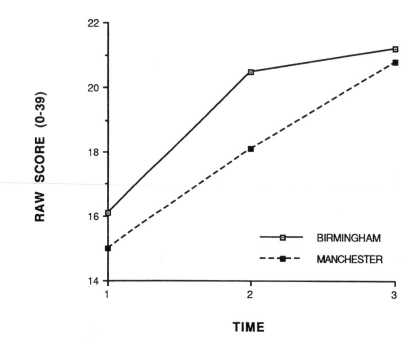

TIME

	TIME 1	TIME 2	TIME 3
BIRMINGHAM			
N	18	19	19
MEAN	16.1	20.5	21.2
SD	6.0	6.1	8.2
MANCHESTER			
N	17	17	17
MEAN	15.0	18.1	20.8
SD	5.0	6.4	7.7

SOURCE OF VARIATION	SUM OF SQUARES	df	Var. Est.	F	Sig.
GROUP	68.27	1,33	68.27	0.61	ns
TIME	598.75	2,66	299.37	31.21	<0.001
GROUP X TIME	25.41	2,66	12.71	1.32	ns

TIME 1 vs TIME 2, t=-6.06, df=34, p<0.001;
TIME 2 vs TIME 3, t=-2.43, df=35, p<0.05.

Figure 6.6 (6.2.3.1)   Pictorial Test of Intelligence: Immediate Recall (Direct Test)

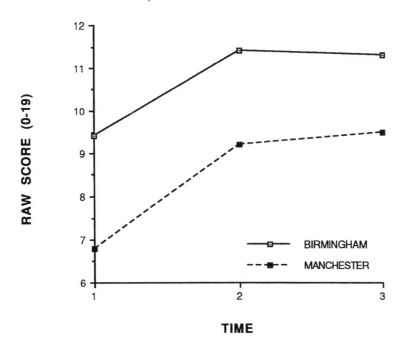

TIME

	TIME 1	TIME 2	TIME 3
BIRMINGHAM			
N	19	19	19
MEAN	9.4	11.4	11.3
SD	3.7	2.8	2.6
MANCHESTER			
N	17	17	17
MEAN	6.8	9.2	9.5
SD	4.2	4.3	5.0

SOURCE OF VARIATION	SUM OF SQUARES	df	Var. Est.	F	Sig.
GROUP	127.26	1,34	127.26	3.77	ns
TIME	126.35	2,68	63.18	13.22	<0.001
GROUP X TIME	3.02	2,68	1.51	0.32	ns

TIME 1 vs TIME 2, t=-4.17, df=35, p<0.001;
TIME 2 vs TIME 3, t=-0.27, df=35, ns.

Figure 6.7 (6.2.3.2)   Pictorial Test of Intelligence: Form Discrimination
(Direct Test)

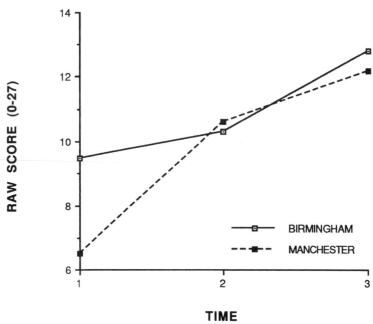

	TIME 1	TIME 2	TIME 3
BIRMINGHAM			
N	19	19	19
MEAN	9.5	10.3	12.8
SD	3.5	4.3	5.5
MANCHESTER			
N	17	17	17
MEAN	6.5	10.6	12.2
SD	5.0	6.8	7.0

SOURCE OF VARIATION	SUM OF SQUARES	df	Var. Est.	F	Sig.
GROUP	32.15	1,34	32.15	0.45	ns
TIME	370.74	2,68	185.37	21.81	<0.001
GROUP X TIME	56.26	2,68	28.13	3.31	<0.05

TIME 1 vs TIME 2, t=-2.80, df=35, p<0.01;
TIME 2 vs TIME 3, t=-3.62, df=35, p<0.01.

174

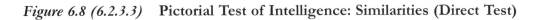

Figure 6.8 (6.2.3.3)   Pictorial Test of Intelligence: Similarities (Direct Test)

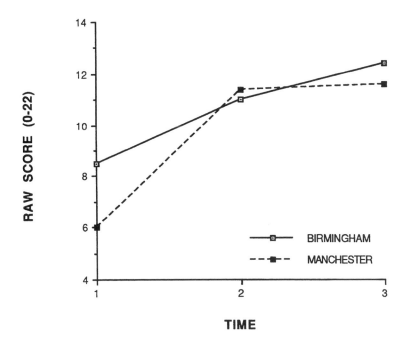

	TIME 1	TIME 2	TIME 3
BIRMINGHAM			
N	19	19	19
MEAN	8.5	11.0	12.4
SD	3.5	4.4	5.1
MANCHESTER			
N	17	17	17
MEAN	6.0	11.4	11.6
SD	3.8	5.0	5.8

GROUP OF VARIATION	SUM OF SQUARES	df	Var. Est.	F	Sig.
GROUP	24.16	1,34	24.16	0.49	ns
TIME	464.54	2,68	232.27	29.70	<0.001
GROUP X TIME	37.73	2,68	18.86	2.41	ns

TIME 1 vs TIME 2, t=-5.10, df=35, p<0.001;
TIME 2 vs TIME 3, t=-1.43, df=35, ns.

Figure 6.9 (6.2.3.4)   Pictorial Test of Intelligence: Information and Comprehension (Direct Test)

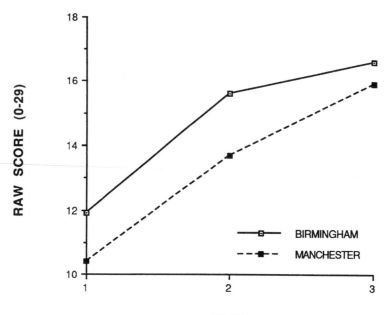

TIME

	TIME 1	TIME 2	TIME 3
BIRMINGHAM			
N	19	19	19
MEAN	11.9	15.6	16.6
SD	4.3	4.0	4.0
MANCHESTER			
N	17	17	17
MEAN	10.4	13.7	15.9
SD	5.9	5.3	7.5

SOURCE OF VARIATION	SUM OF SQUARES	df	Var. Est.	F	Sig.
GROUP	51.55	1,34	51.55	0.80	ns
TIME	488.93	2,68	244.47	26.77	<0.001
GROUP X TIME	7.16	2,68	3.58	0.39	ns

TIME 1 vs TIME 2, t=-4.70, df=35, p<0.001;
TIME 2 vs TIME 3, t=-2.67, df=35, p<0.05.

Figure 6.10 (6.2.3.5)   Pictorial Test of Intelligence: Size and Number (Direct Test)

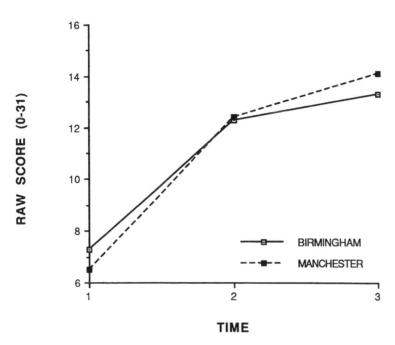

	TIME 1	TIME 2	TIME 3
BIRMINGHAM			
N	19	19	19
MEAN	7.3	12.3	13.3
SD	3.5	5.0	5.8
MANCHESTER			
N	17	17	17
MEAN	6.5	12.4	14.1
SD	5.0	6.4	6.9

SOURCE OF VARIATION	SUM OF SQUARES	df	Var Est.	F	Sig.
GROUP	0.07	1,34	0.07	0.00	ns
TIME	919.70	2,68	459.85	45.36	<0.001
GROUP X TIME	10.51	2,68	5.26	0.52	ns

TIME 1 vs TIME 2, t=-7.44, df=35, p<0.001;
TIME 2 vs TIME 3, t=-1.89, df=35, ns.

177

Figure 6.11 (6.2.3.6)   Pictorial Test of Intelligence: Picture Vocabulary
(Direct Test)

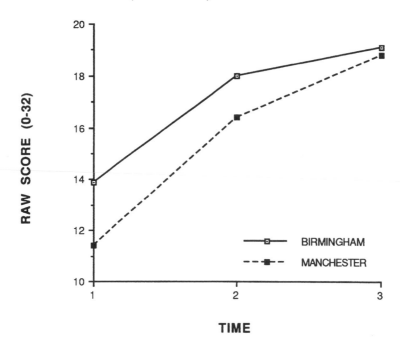

	TIME 1	TIME 2	TIME 3
BIRMINGHAM			
N	19	19	19
MEAN	13.9	18.0	19.1
SD	5.6	4.0	4.4
MANCHESTER			
N	17	17	17
MEAN	11.4	16.4	18.8
SD	6.7	5.7	8.2

SOURCE OF VARIATION	SUM OF SQUARES	df	Var. Est.	F	Sig.
GROUP	59.61	1,34	59.61	0.74	ns
TIME	762.24	2,68	381.12	33.48	<0.001
GROUP X TIME	24.13	2,68	12.06	1.06	ns

TIME 1 vs TIME 2, t=-5.46, df=35, p<0.001;
TIME 2 vs TIME 3, t=-2.10, df=35, p<0.05.

Figure 6.12 (6.2.3.7)   Pictorial Test of Intelligence: General Cognition
(Direct Test)

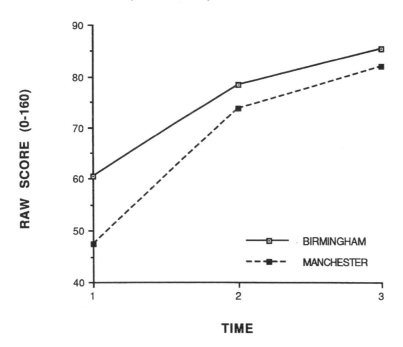

	TIME 1	TIME 2	TIME 3
BIRMINGHAM			
N	19	19	19
MEAN	60.5	78.5	85.5
SD	17.2	18.7	22.5
MANCHESTER			
N	17	17	17
MEAN	47.5	73.8	82.2
SD	27.3	28.9	37.4

SOURCE OF VARIATION	SUM OF SQUARES	df	Var Est.	F	Sig.
GROUP	1332.56	1,34	1332.56	0.73	ns
TIME	17202.91	2,68	8601.45	88.46	<0.001
GROUP X TIME	487.13	2,68	243.56	2.50	ns

TIME 1 vs TIME 2, t=-8.91, df=35, p<0.001;
TIME 2 vs TIME 3, t=-3.97, df=35, p<0.001.

Figure 6.13 (6.2.4.1)   Achievement Test: Reading (Direct Test)

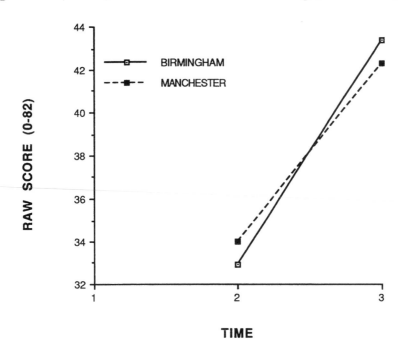

	TIME 1	TIME 2	TIME 3
BIRMINGHAM			
N		19	19
MEAN		32.9	43.4
SD		16.9	21.7
MANCHESTER			
N		17	17
MEAN		34.0	42.3
SD		19.9	24.8

SOURCE OF VARIATION	SUM OF SQUARES	df	Var. Est.	F	Sig.
GROUP	0.00	1,34	0.00	0.00	ns
TIME	1571.29	1,34	1571.29	24.38	<0.001
GROUP X TIME	20.29	1,34	20.29	0.31	ns

Figure 6.14 (6.2.4.2)   Achievement Test: Mathematics (Direct Test)

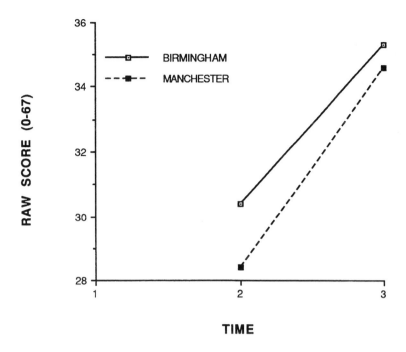

	TIME 1	TIME 2	TIME 3
BIRMINGHAM			
N		19	19
MEAN		30.4	35.2
SD		12.4	15.5
MANCHESTER			
N		17	17
MEAN		28.4	34.6
SD		15.3	16.9

SOURCE OF VARIATION	SUM OF SQUARES	df	Var. Est.	F	Sig.
GROUP	31.07	1,34	31.07	0.07	ns
TIME	549.87	1,34	549.87	20.98	<0.001
GROUP X TIME	7.37	1,34	7.37	0.28	ns

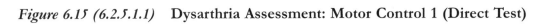

Figure 6.15 (6.2.5.1.1)   Dysarthria Assessment: Motor Control 1 (Direct Test)

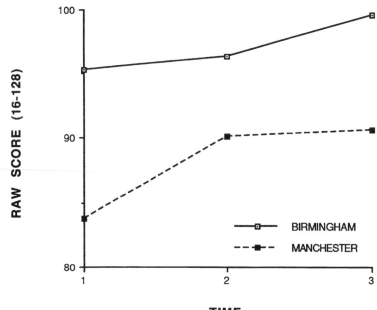

	TIME 1	TIME 2	TIME 3
BIRMINGHAM			
N	18	19	19
MEAN	95.3	96.3	99.6
SD	26.4	26.4	25.8
MANCHESTER			
N	17	17	17
MEAN	83.8	90.1	90.6
SD	30.6	29.6	28.1

SOURCE OF VARIATION	SUM OF SQUARES	df	Var. Est.	F	Sig.
GROUP	2721.25	1,33	2721.25	1.23	ns
TIME	800.84	2,66	400.42	10.73	<0.001
GROUP X TIME	63.53	2,66	31.76	0.85	ns

TIME 1 vs TIME 2, t=-3.65, df=34, p<0.01;
TIME 2 vs TIME 3, t=-1.60, df=35, ns.

Figure 6.16 (6.2.5.1.2)   Dysarthria Assessment: Motor Control 2 (Direct Test)

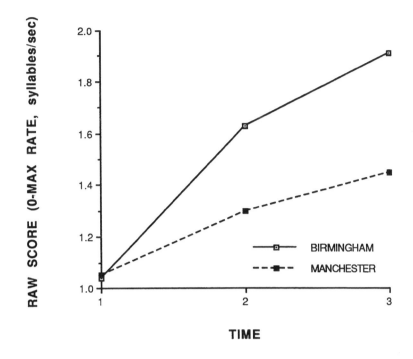

	TIME 1	TIME 2	TIME 3
BIRMINGHAM			
N	18	19	18
MEAN	1.04	1.63	1.91
SD	1.00	1.25	1.21
MANCHESTER			
N	17	17	15
MEAN	1.05	1.30	1.45
SD	0.92	0.97	1.16

SOURCE OF VARIATION	SUM OF SQUARES	df	Var. Est.	F	Sig.
GROUP	4.94	1,30	4.94	1.62	ns
TIME	8.24	2,60	4.12	25.18	<0.001
GROUP X TIME	0.98	2,60	0.49	2.99	ns

TIME 1 vs TIME 2, t=-4.25, df=34, p<0.001;
TIME 2 vs TIME 3, t=-2.86, df=32, p<0.01.

Figure 6.17 (6.2.5.2.1)   Preverbal Communication: Motor Control 3 (Direct Test)

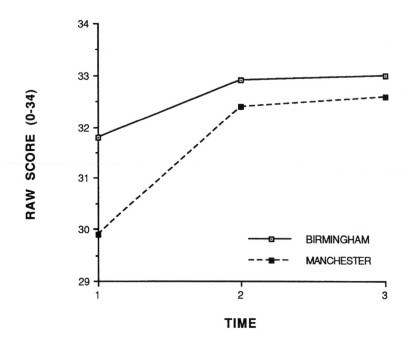

	TIME 1	TIME 2	TIME 3
BIRMINGHAM			
N	18	19	19
MEAN	31.8	32.9	33.0
SD	6.3	3.3	3.0
MANCHESTER			
N	17	17	17
MEAN	29.9	32.4	32.6
SD	9.3	5.4	5.8

SOURCE OF VARIATION	SUM OF SQUARES	df	Var. Est.	F	Sig.
GROUP	22.65	1,33	22.65	0.27	ns
TIME	77.91	2,66	38.96	3.91	<0.05
GROUP X TIME	13.76	2,66	6.88	0.69	ns

TIME 1 vs TIME 2, t=-1.98, df=34, ns;
TIME 2 vs TIME 3, t=-0.92, df=35, ns.

Figure 6.18 (6.2.5.2.2) Preverbal Communication: Receptive Non-Verbal
(Direct Test)

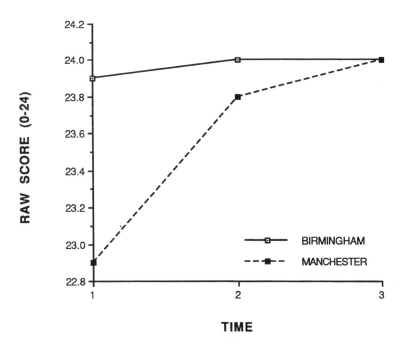

	TIME 1	TIME 2	TIME 3
BIRMINGHAM			
N	18	19	19
MEAN	23.9	24.0	24.0
SD	0.5	0.0	0.0
MANCHESTER			
N	17	17	17
MEAN	22.9	23.8	24.0
SD	4.6	0.7	0.0

SOURCE OF VARIATION	SUM OF SQUARES	df	Var. Est.	F	Sig.
GROUP	4.08	1,33	4.08	0.88	ns
TIME	7.72	2,66	3.86	1.28	ns
GROUP X TIME	5.05	2,66	2.53	0.84	ns

TIME 1 vs TIME 2, t=-1.12, df=34, ns;
TIME 2 vs TIME 3, t=-1.00, df=35, ns.

185

Figure 6.19 (6.2.5.2.3)   Preverbal Communication: Expressive Non-Verbal
(Direct Test)

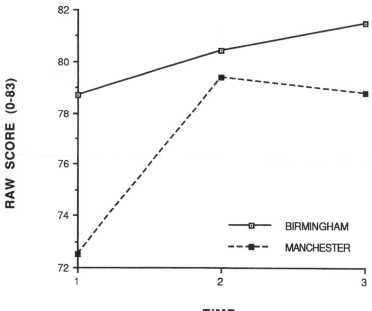

	TIME 1	TIME 2	TIME 3
BIRMINGHAM			
N	18	19	19
MEAN	78.7	80.4	81.5
SD	11.5	7.8	5.0
MANCHESTER			
N	17	17	17
MEAN	72.5	79.4	78.8
SD	24.3	11.6	16.0

SOURCE OF VARIATION	SUM OF SQUARES	df	Var. Est.	F	Sig.
GROUP	279.74	1,33	279.74	0.62	ns
TIME	448.10	2,66	224.05	3.22	<0.05
GROUP X TIME	131.30	2,66	65.65	0.94	ns

TIME 1 vs TIME 2, t=-1.84, df=34, ns;
TIME 2 vs TIME 3, t=-0.40, df=35, ns.

Figure 6.20 (6.2.5.2.4)   Preverbal Communication: Receptive Verbal (Direct Test)

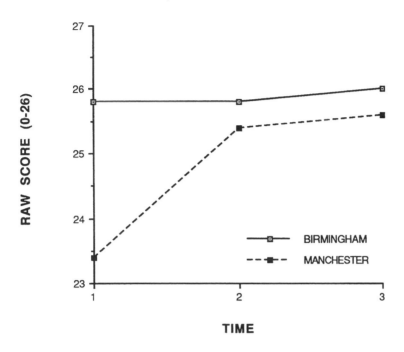

TIME

	TIME 1	TIME 2	TIME 3
BIRMINGHAM			
N	18	19	19
MEAN	25.8	25.8	26.0
SD	0.7	0.7	0.0
MANCHESTER			
N	17	17	17
MEAN	23.4	25.4	25.6
SD	5.9	2.0	1.1

SOURCE OF VARIATION	SUM OF SQUARES	df	Var. Est.	F	Sig.
GROUP	27.74	1,33	27.74	2.45	ns
TIME	29.87	2,66	14.93	3.59	<0.05
GROUP X TIME	23.47	2,66	11.73	2.82	ns

TIME 1 vs TIME 2, t=-1.86, df=34, ns;
TIME 2 vs TIME 3, t=-1.14, df=35, ns.

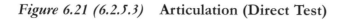

Figure 6.21 (6.2.5.3)   Articulation (Direct Test)

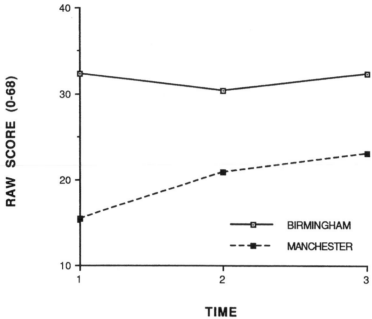

TIME

	TIME 1	TIME 2	TIME 3
BIRMINGHAM			
N	18	19	19
MEAN	32.3	30.4	32.3
SD	20.1	18.6	18.0
MANCHESTER			
N	17	17	17
MEAN	15.4	20.9	23.1
SD	13.6	17.9	17.7

SOURCE OF VARIATION	SUM OF SQUARES	df	Var. Est.	F	Sig.
GROUP	4241.59	1,33	4241.59	4.95	<0.05
TIME	345.81	2,66	172.91	4.33	<0.05
GROUP X TIME	233.13	2,66	116.56	2.92	ns

TIME 1 vs TIME 2, t=-1.45, df=34, ns;
TIME 2 vs TIME 3, t=-2.60, df=35, p<0.05.

188

Figure 6.22 (6.2.5.4)   Expressive Verbal (Direct Test)

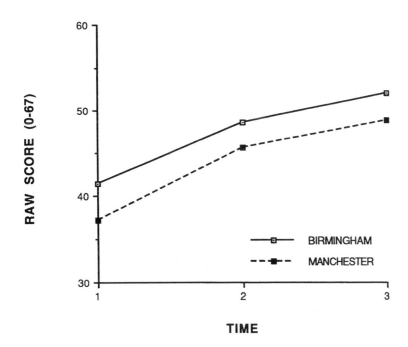

	TIME 1	TIME 2	TIME 3
BIRMINGHAM			
N	18	19	19
MEAN	41.4	48.4	52.0
SD	14.8	15.0	14.9
MANCHESTER			
N	17	17	17
MEAN	37.2	45.6	48.8
SD	15.8	14.7	15.2

SOURCE OF VARIATION	SUM OF SQUARES	df	Var. Est.	F	Sig.
GROUP	292.76	1,33	292.76	0.45	ns
TIME	2236.19	2,66	1118.10	60.25	<0.001
GROUP X TIME	11.89	2,66	5.94	0.32	ns

TIME 1 vs TIME 2, t=-7.31, df=34, p<0.001;
TIME 2 vs TIME 3, t=-4.52, df=35, p<0.001.

189

Figure 6.23 (6.2.6.1)   Fine Motor Assessment: Fine Motor Independence
(Direct Test)

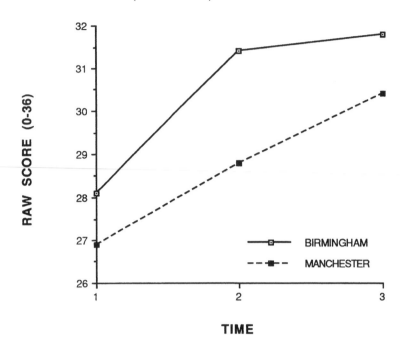

	TIME 1	TIME 2	TIME 3
BIRMINGHAM			
N	19	19	19
MEAN	28.1	31.4	31.8
SD	8.4	5.7	5.3
MANCHESTER			
N	17	17	17
MEAN	26.9	28.8	30.4
SD	10.1	9.2	7.9

SOURCE OF VARIATION	SUM OF SQUARES	df	Var. Est.	F	Sig.
GROUP	82.65	1,34	82.65	0.50	ns
TIME	248.36	2,68	124.18	10.97	<0.001
GROUP X TIME	8.77	2,68	4.39	0.39	ns

TIME 1 vs TIME 2, t=-2.97, df=35, p<0.01;
TIME 2 vs TIME 3, t=-1.76, df=35, ns.

Figure 6.24 (6.2.6.2)   Fine Motor Assessment: Object Transfer 1 (Direct Test)

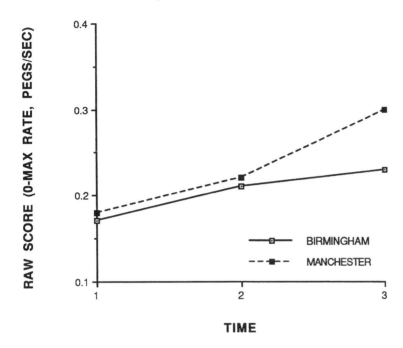

TIME

	TIME 1	TIME 2	TIME 3
BIRMINGHAM			
N	19	19	19
MEAN	0.17	0.21	0.23
SD	0.11	0.11	0.11
MANCHESTER			
N	17	17	17
MEAN	0.18	0.22	0.30
SD	0.10	0.11	0.20

SOURCE OF VARIATION	SUM OF SQUARES	df	Var. Est.	F	Sig.
GROUP	0.022	1,34	0.022	0.51	ns
TIME	0.152	2,68	0.076	24.92	<0.001
GROUP X TIME	0.023	2,68	0.012	3.79	<0.05

TIME 1 vs TIME 2, t=-4.65, df=35, p<0.001;
TIME 2 vs TIME 3, t=-3.65, df=35, p<0.05.

Figure 6.25 (6.2.6.3)   Fine Motor Assessment: Object Transfer 2 (Direct Test)

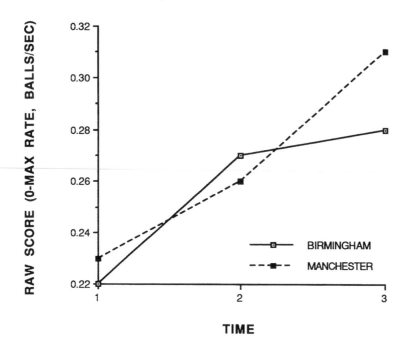

	TIME 1	TIME 2	TIME 3
BIRMINGHAM			
N	19	19	19
MEAN	0.22	0.27	0.28
SD	0.12	0.13	0.14
MANCHESTER			
N	17	17	17
MEAN	0.23	0.26	0.31
SD	0.17	0.14	0.21

SOURCE OF VARIATION	SUM OF SQUARES	df	Var. Est.	F	Sig.
GROUP	0.002	1,34	0.002	0.03	ns
TIME	0.085	2,68	0.043	8.45	<0.05
GROUP X TIME	0.009	2,68	0.005	0.98	ns

TIME 1 vs TIME 2, t=-2.13, df=35, p<0.05;
TIME 2 vs TIME 3, t=-1.84, df=35, ns.

Figure 6.26 (6.2.6.4)   Fine Motor Assessment: Manipulation (Direct Test)

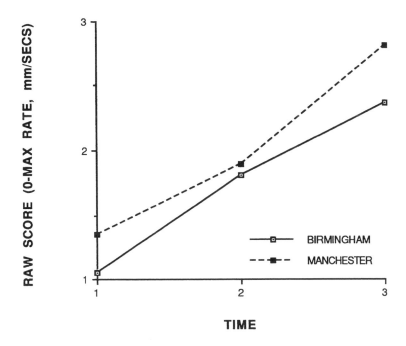

	TIME 1	TIME 2	TIME 3
BIRMINGHAM			
N	19	19	19
MEAN	1.05	1.81	2.37
SD	0.68	1.11	1.71
MANCHESTER			
N	17	17	17
MEAN	1.35	1.90	2.81
SD	1.08	1.61	2.42

SOURCE OF VARIATION	SUM OF SQUARES	df	Var. Est.	F	Sig.
GROUP	2.03	1,34	2.03	0.38	ns
TIME	34.79	2,68	17.40	22.72	<0.001
GROUP X TIME	0.57	2,68	0.28	0.36	ns

TIME 1 vs TIME 2, t=-4.05, df=35, p<0.001;
TIME 2 vs TIME 3, t=-3.58, df=35, p<0.05.

Figure 6.27 (6.2.6.5)   Fine Motor Assessment: Two Hand Coordination
(Direct Test)

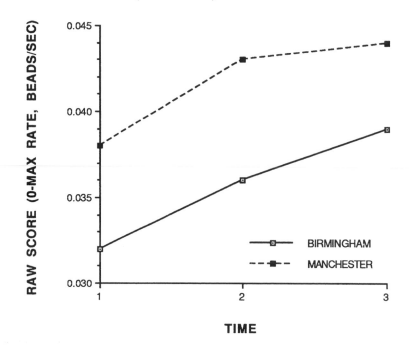

	TIME 1	TIME 2	TIME 3
BIRMINGHAM			
N	19	19	19
MEAN	0.032	0.036	0.039
SD	0.014	0.013	0.016
MANCHESTER			
N	17	17	17
MEAN	0.038	0.043	0.044
SD	0.018	0.013	0.025

SOURCE OF VARIATION	SUM OF SQUARES	df	Var. Est.	F	Sig.
GROUP	0.0009	1,34	0.0009	1.44	ns
TIME	0.0008	2,68	0.0004	3.84	<0.05
GROUP X TIME	0.0000	2,68	0.0000	0.06	ns

TIME 1 vs TIME 2, t=-1.95, df=35, ns;
TIME 2 vs TIME 3, t=-0.57, df=35, ns.

Figure 6.28 (6.2.6.6)   Fine Motor Assessment: Pen Placement (Direct Test)

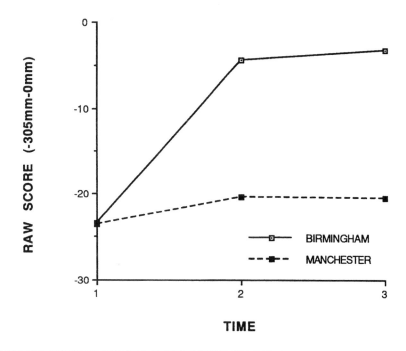

	TIME 1	TIME 2	TIME 3
BIRMINGHAM			
N	19	19	19
MEAN	-23.5	-4.3	-3.2
SD	70.2	4.0	2.1
MANCHESTER			
N	17	17	17
MEAN	-23.6	-20.4	-20.5
SD	72.9	73.4	73.4

SOURCE OF VARIATION	SUM OF SQUARES	df	Var. Est.	F	Sig.
GROUP	3342.66	1,34	3342.66	0.39	ns
TIME	3128.96	2,68	1564.48	1.84	ns
GROUP X TIME	1647.28	2,68	823.64	0.97	ns

TIME 1 vs TIME 2, t=-1.41, df=35, ns;
TIME 2 vs TIME 3, t=-0.91, df=35, ns.

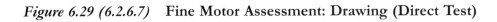

Figure 6.29 (6.2.6.7)   Fine Motor Assessment: Drawing (Direct Test)

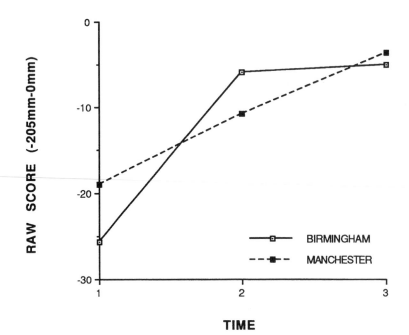

	TIME 1	TIME 2	TIME 3
BIRMINGHAM			
N	19	19	19
MEAN	-25.6	-5.9	-5.0
SD	55.5	5.1	5.3
MANCHESTER			
N	17	17	17
MEAN	-19.0	-10.8	-3.6
SD	48.5	26.7	4.2

SOURCE OF VARIATION	SUM OF SQUARES	df	Var. Est.	F	Sig.
GROUP	27.56	1,34	27.56	0.02	ns
TIME	6409.08	2,68	3204.54	4.22	<0.05
GROUP X TIME	590.70	2,68	295.35	0.39	ns

TIME 1 vs TIME 2, t=-2.04, df=35, p<0.05;
TIME 2 vs TIME 3, t=-1.45, df=35, ns.

Figure 6.30 (6.2.7.1)   Gross Motor Assessment: Postural Independence
(Direct Test)

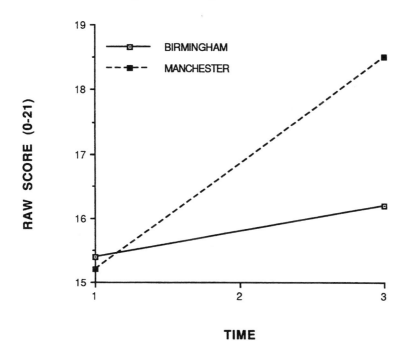

	TIME 1	TIME 2	TIME 3
BIRMINGHAM			
N	19		19
MEAN	15.4		16.2
SD	3.9		3.8
MANCHESTER			
N	17		17
MEAN	15.2		18.5
SD	5.3		3.0

SOURCE OF VARIATION	SUM OF SQUARES	df	Var. Est.	F	Sig.
GROUP	18.22	1,34	18.22	0.63	ns
TIME	74.81	1,34	74.81	19.51	<0.001
GROUP X TIME	28.14	1,34	28.14	7.34	<0.05

Figure 6.31 (6.2.7.2)   Gross Motor Assessment: Position Changing
Independence (Direct Test)

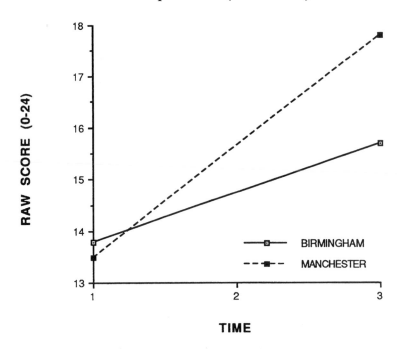

	TIME 1	TIME 2	TIME 3
BIRMINGHAM			
N	19		19
MEAN	13.8		15.7
SD	5.4		5.5
MANCHESTER			
N	17		17
MEAN	13.5		17.8
SD	7.2		5.1

SOURCE OF VARIATION	SUM OF SQUARES	df	Var. Est.	F	Sig.
GROUP	13.10	1,34	13.10	0.21	ns
TIME	174.76	1,34	174.76	32.08	<0.001
GROUP X TIME	24.71	1,34	24.71	4.53	<0.05

Figure 6.32 (6.2.7.6)   Gross Motor Assessment: Locomotion Independence
(Direct Test)

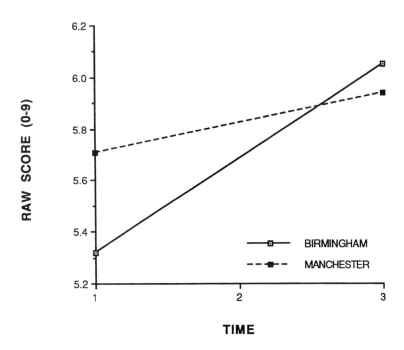

	TIME 1	TIME 2	TIME 3
BIRMINGHAM			
N	19		19
MEAN	5.3		6.1
SD	2.2		2.3
MANCHESTER			
N	17		16
MEAN	5.7		5.9
SD	2.7		2.8

SOURCE OF VARIATION	SUM OF SQUARES	df	Var. Est.	F	Sig.
GROUP	0.16	1,33	0.16	0.01	ns
TIME	4.78	1,33	4.78	6.17	<0.05
GROUP X TIME	0.78	1,33	0.78	1.01	ns

Figure 6.33 (6.2.7.7) Gross Motor Assessment: Position Changing (Direct Test)

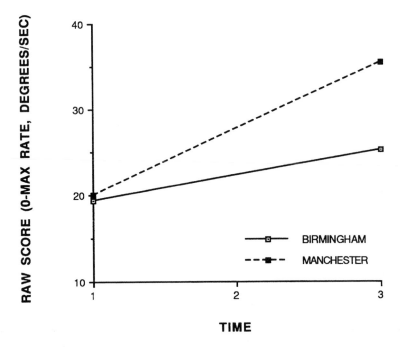

	TIME 1	TIME 2	TIME 3
BIRMINGHAM			
N	19		19
MEAN	19.3		25.2
SD	13.4		16.3
MANCHESTER			
N	17		17
MEAN	20.0		35.5
SD	14.4		18.6

SOURCE OF VARIATION	SUM OF SQUARES	df	Var. Est.	F	Sig.
GROUP	541.14	1,34	541.14	1.37	ns
TIME	2040.40	1,34	2040.40	20.02	<0.001
GROUP X TIME	411.66	1,34	411.66	4.04	ns

Figure 6.34 (6.2.7.8)   Gross Motor Assessment: Crawling (Direct Test)

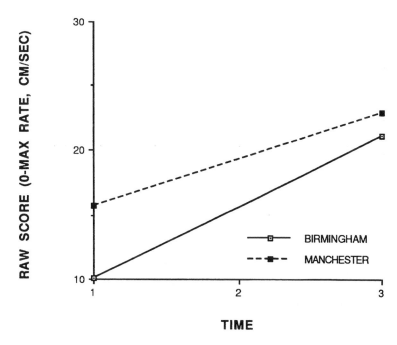

	TIME 1	TIME 2	TIME 3
BIRMINGHAM			
N	19		19
MEAN	10.1		21.1
SD	20.7		30.8
MANCHESTER			
N	17		16
MEAN	15.7		22.9
SD	22.3		29.5

SOURCE OF VARIATION	SUM OF SQUARES	df	Var. Est.	F	Sig.
GROUP	236.06	1,33	236.06	0.20	ns
TIME	1445.77	1,33	1445.77	7.47	<0.05
GROUP X TIME	60.53	1,33	60.53	0.31	ns

Figure 6.35 (6.2.7.9)   Gross Motor Assessment: Walking (Direct Test)

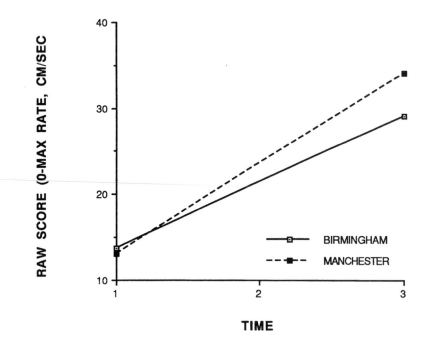

	TIME 1	TIME 2	TIME 3
BIRMINGHAM			
N	19		19
MEAN	13.7		29.1
SD	14.7		34.7
MANCHESTER			
N	17		17
MEAN	13.1		34.1
SD	12.8		39.8

SOURCE OF VARIATION	SUM OF SQUARES	df	Var. Est.	F	Sig.
GROUP	86.91	1,34	86.91	0.07	ns
TIME	5944.22	1,34	5944.22	15.44	<0.001
GROUP X TIME	146.61	1,34	146.61	0.38	ns

Figure 6.36 (6.2.7.10)   Gross Motor Assessment: Preferred Locomotion
(Direct Test)

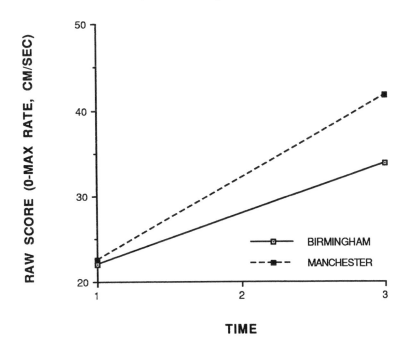

	TIME 1	TIME 2	TIME 3
BIRMINGHAM			
N	19		19
MEAN	22.1		33.9
SD	23.1		34.2
MANCHESTER			
N	17		17
MEAN	22.6		41.8
SD	21.8		37.1

SOURCE OF VARIATION	SUM OF SQUARES	df	Var. Est.	F	Sig.
GROUP	317.85	1,34	317.85	0.21	ns
TIME	4302.89	1,34	4302.89	16.55	<0.001
GROUP X TIME	250.00	1,34	250.00	0.96	ns

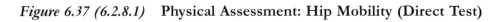

Figure 6.37 (6.2.8.1)   Physical Assessment: Hip Mobility (Direct Test)

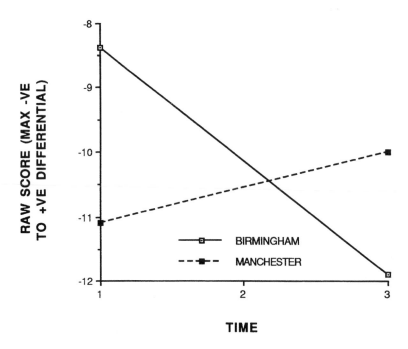

TIME

	TIME 1	TIME 2	TIME 3
BIRMINGHAM			
N	19		19
MEAN	-8.4		-11.9
SD	6.5		4.6
MANCHESTER			
N	17		17
MEAN	-11.1		-10.0
SD	8.0		7.3

SOURCE OF VARIATION	SUM OF SQUARES	df	Var. Est.	F	Sig.
GROUP	3.24	1,34	3.24	0.05	ns
TIME	24.93	1,34	24.93	1.33	ns
GROUP X TIME	97.56	1,34	97.56	5.22	<0.05

Figure 6.38 (6.2.8.2)   Physical Assessment: Hamstring Extensibility (Direct Test)

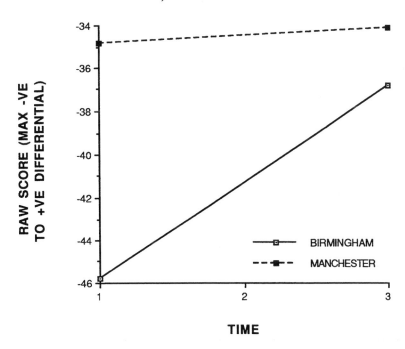

TIME

	TIME 1	TIME 2	TIME 3
BIRMINGHAM			
N	19		19
MEAN	-45.7		-36.8
SD	11.1		16.8
MANCHESTER			
N	17		17
MEAN	-34.8		-34.1
SD	18.4		21.5

SOURCE OF VARIATION	SUM OF SQUARES	df	Var. Est.	F	Sig.
GROUP	830.66	1,34	830.66	1.77	ns
TIME	415.90	1,34	415.90	3.37	ns
GROUP X TIME	308.10	1,34	308.10	2.49	ns

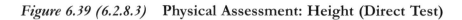

Figure 6.39 (6.2.8.3)   Physical Assessment: Height (Direct Test)

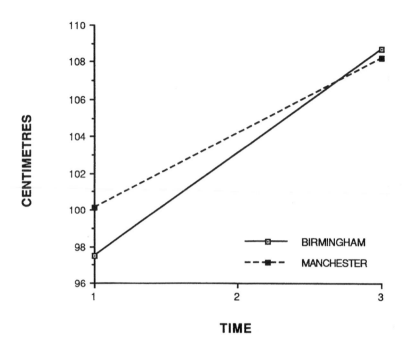

	TIME 1	TIME 2	TIME 3
BIRMINGHAM			
N	19		19
MEAN	97.5		108.7
SD	5.5		6.0
MANCHESTER			
N	17		17
MEAN	100.1		108.2
SD	8.6		6.3

SOURCE OF VARIATION	SUM OF SQUARES	df	Var. Est.	F	Sig.
GROUP	20.27	1,34	20.27	0.26	ns
TIME	1691.63	1,34	1691.63	153.88	<0.001
GROUP X TIME	42.16	1,34	42.16	3.84	ns

Figure 6.40 (6.2.8.4)   Physical Assessment: Weight (Direct Test)

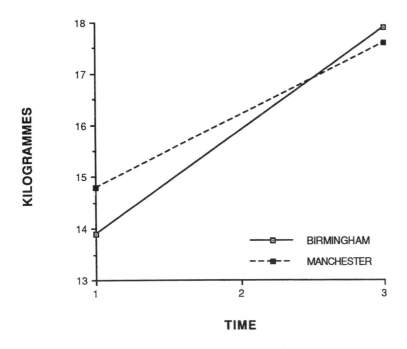

TIME

	TIME 1	TIME 2	TIME 3
BIRMINGHAM			
N	19		19
MEAN	13.9		17.9
SD	1.8		4.7
MANCHESTER			
N	17		17
MEAN	14.8		17.6
SD	2.0		3.4

SOURCE OF VARIATION	SUM OF SQUARES	df	Var. Est.	F	Sig.
GROUP	1.33	1,34	1.33	0.08	ns
TIME	205.10	1,34	205.10	58.13	<0.001
GROUP X TIME	7.48	1,34	7.48	2.12	ns

Figure 6.41 (6.2.8.5)   Physical Assessment: Neurology (Direct Test)

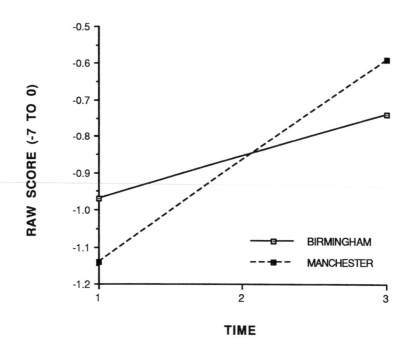

TIME

	TIME 1	TIME 2	TIME 3
BIRMINGHAM			
N	19		19
MEAN	-0.97		-0.74
SD	0.98		0.81
MANCHESTER			
N	17		17
MEAN	-1.14		-0.59
SD	1.22		0.87

SOURCE OF VARIATION	SUM OF SQUARES	df	Var. Est.	F	Sig.
GROUP	0.00	1,34	0.00	0.00	ns
TIME	2.76	1,34	2.76	4.41	<0.05
GROUP X TIME	0.43	1,34	0.43	0.69	ns

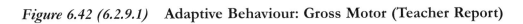
Figure 6.42 (6.2.9.1)   Adaptive Behaviour: Gross Motor (Teacher Report)

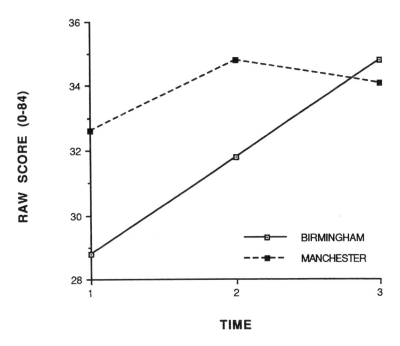

	TIME 1	TIME 2	TIME 3
BIRMINGHAM			
N	19	19	19
MEAN	28.8	31.8	34.8
SD	14.3	15.7	18.6
MANCHESTER			
N	17	17	17
MEAN	32.6	34.8	34.1
SD	18.7	21.8	22.7

SOURCE OF VARIATION	SUM OF SQUARES	df	Var. Est.	F	Sig.
GROUP	107.56	1,34	107.56	0.11	ns
TIME	257.49	2,68	128.75	4.58	<0.05
GROUP X TIME	107.27	2,68	53.63	1.91	ns

TIME 1 vs TIME 2, t=-2.09, df=35, p<0.05;
TIME 2 vs TIME 3, t=-1.06, df=35, ns.

Figure 6.43 (6.2.9.2) Adaptive Behaviour: Interpersonal (Teacher Report)

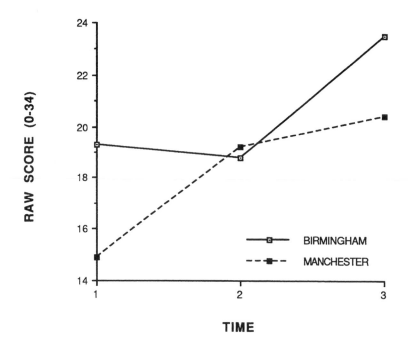

TIME

	TIME 1	TIME 2	TIME 3
BIRMINGHAM			
N	19	19	19
MEAN	19.3	18.8	23.5
SD	5.8	6.4	4.7
MANCHESTER			
N	17	17	17
MEAN	14.9	19.2	20.4
SD	7.3	5.8	6.5

SOURCE OF VARIATION	SUM OF SQUARES	df	Var. Est.	F	Sig.
GROUP	151.12	1,34	151.12	1.84	ns
TIME	421.73	2,68	210.87	14.00	<0.001
GROUP X TIME	114.40	2,68	57.20	3.80	<0.05

TIME 1 vs TIME 2, t=-1.86, df=35, ns;
TIME 2 vs TIME 3, t=-3.22, df=35, p<0.01.

Figure 6.44 (6.2.9.3)   Adaptive Behaviour: Play (Teacher Report)

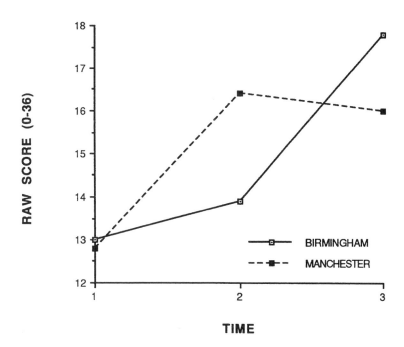

	TIME 1	TIME 2	TIME 3
BIRMINGHAM			
N	19	19	19
MEAN	13.0	13.9	17.8
SD	3.9	3.9	4.5
MANCHESTER			
N	17	17	17
MEAN	12.8	16.4	16.0
SD	4.4	4.1	4.4

SOURCE OF VARIATION	SUM OF SQUARES	df	Var. Est.	F	Sig.
GROUP	0.58	1,34	0.58	0.02	ns
TIME	286.13	2,68	143.07	19.19	<0.001
GROUP X TIME	80.35	2,68	40.18	5.39	<0.01

TIME 1 vs TIME 2, t=-3.67, df=35, p<0.01;
TIME 2 vs TIME 3, t=-2.53, df=35, p<0.05.

Figure 6.45 (6.2.9.4)   Adaptive Behaviour: Activities of Daily Living (Teacher Report)

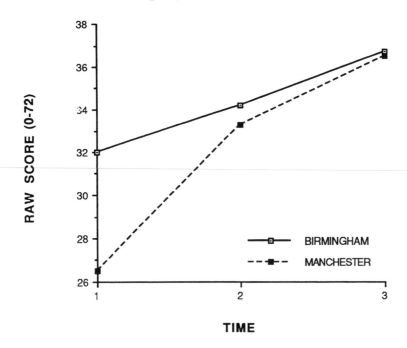

TIME

	TIME 1	TIME 2	TIME 3
BIRMINGHAM			
N	19	19	19
MEAN	32.0	34.2	36.7
SD	11.4	12.0	10.3
MANCHESTER			
N	17	17	17
MEAN	26.5	33.3	36.5
SD	10.8	11.6	13.0

SOURCE OF VARIATION	SUM OF SQUARES	df	Var. Est.	F	Sig.
GROUP	132.39	1,34	132.39	0.37	ns
TIME	982.52	2,68	491.26	25.38	<0.001
GROUP X TIME	144.30	2,68	72.15	3.73	<0.05

TIME 1 vs TIME 2, t=-5.21, df=35, p<0.001;
TIME 2 vs TIME 3, t=-2.78, df=35, p<0.01.

Figure 6.46 (6.2.9.5)   Adaptive Behaviour: Attention and Control (Teacher
Report)

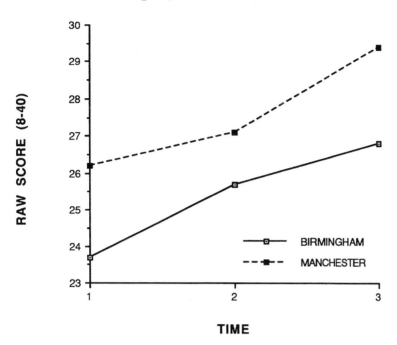

	TIME 1	TIME 2	TIME 3
BIRMINGHAM			
N	19	19	19
MEAN	23.7	25.7	26.8
SD	5.6	4.6	6.7
MANCHESTER			
N	17	17	17
MEAN	26.2	27.1	29.4
SD	6.9	7.2	6.7

SOURCE OF VARIATION	SUM OF SQUARES	df	Var. Est.	F	Sig.
GROUP	123.90	1,34	123.90	1.39	ns
TIME	180.68	2,68	90.34	5.88	<0.01
GROUP X TIME	9.20	2,68	4.60	0.30	ns

TIME 1 vs TIME 2, t=-2.31, df=35, p<0.05;
TIME 2 vs TIME 3, t=-1.67, df=35, ns.

Figure 6.47 (6.2.10) Behaviour Problems (Mother's Questionnaire)

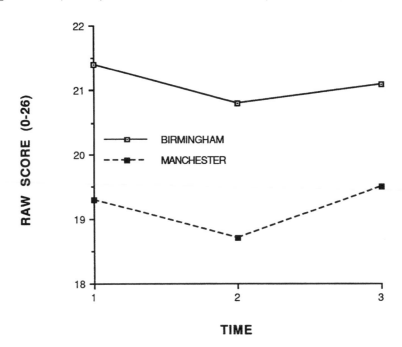

	TIME 1	TIME 2	TIME 3
BIRMINGHAM			
N	19	18	19
MEAN	21.4	20.8	21.1
SD	2.7	3.4	3.6
MANCHESTER			
N	17	15	17
MEAN	19.3	18.7	19.5
SD	3.1	4.2	3.4

SOURCE OF VARIATION	SUM OF SQUARES	df	Var. Est.	F	Sig.
GROUP	72.49	1,31	72.49	2.57	ns
TIME	9.76	2,62	4.88	1.21	ns
GROUP X TIME	2.40	2,62	1.20	0.30	ns

TIME 1 vs TIME 2, t=1.52, df=32, ns;
TIME 2 vs TIME 3, t=-0.99, df=32, ns.

214

Figure 6.48 (6.6.4.1)   Factor 1 Gross-Motor

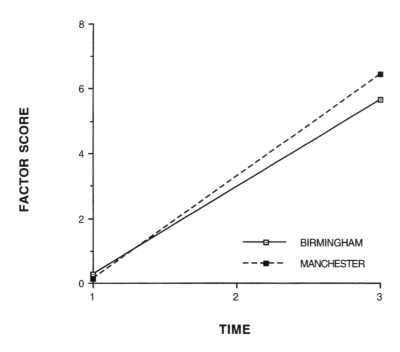

	TIME 1	TIME 2	TIME 3
BIRMINGHAM			
N	18		18
MEAN	0.27		5.68
SD	8.69		11.41
MANCHESTER			
N	17		15
MEAN	0.13		6.45
SD	9.06		12.67

SOURCE OF VARIATION	SUM OF SQUARES	df	Var. Est.	F	Sig.
GROUP	1.04	1,30	1.04	0.00	ns
TIME	797.82	1,30	797.82	84.35	<0.001
GROUP X TIME	2.84	1,30	2.84	0.30	ns

Figure 6.49 (6.6.4.2)   Factor 2 Expressive Language

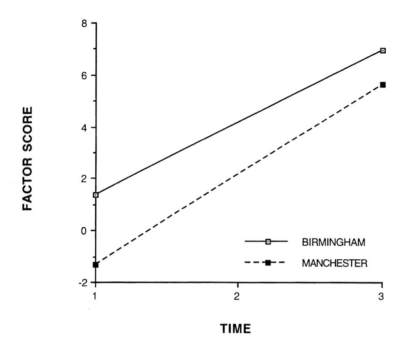

	TIME 1	TIME 2	TIME 3
BIRMINGHAM			
N	18		18
MEAN	1.37		6.99
SD	7.22		7.76
MANCHESTER			
N	17		15
MEAN	-1.32		5.66
SD	8.93		8.73

SOURCE OF VARIATION	SUM OF SQUARES	df	Var. Est.	F	Sig.
GROUP	105.53	1,30	105.53	0.79	ns
TIME	771.02	1,30	771.02	174.37	<0.001
GROUP X TIME	12.34	1,30	12.34	2.79	ns

216

Figure 6.50 (6.6.4.3)   Factor 4 Cognitive and Social

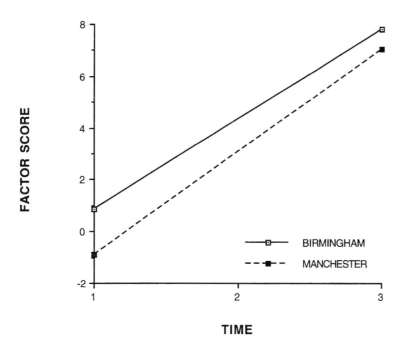

	TIME 1	TIME 2	TIME 3
BIRMINGHAM			
N	18		18
MEAN	0.87		7.84
SD	5.56		6.28
MANCHESTER			
N	17		15
MEAN	-0.87		7.07
SD	7.44		7.96

SOURCE OF VARIATION	SUM OF SQUARES	df	Var. Est.	F	Sig.
GROUP	40.70	1,30	40.70	0.44	ns
TIME	962.79	1,30	962.79	216.62	<0.001
GROUP X TIME	6.23	1,30	6.23	1.40	ns

Figure 6.51 (6.6.4.4)   Factor 5 Independence and Motor

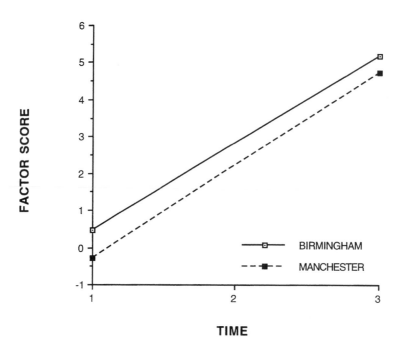

	TIME 1	TIME 2	TIME 3
BIRMINGHAM			
N	18		18
MEAN	0.46		5.18
SD	6.38		7.17
MANCHESTER			
N	17		15
MEAN	-0.28		4.75
SD	7.10		8.47

SOURCE OF VARIATION	SUM OF SQUARES	df	Var. Est.	F	Sig.
GROUP	23.75	1,30	23.75	0.23	ns
TIME	513.88	1,30	513.88	144.78	<0.001
GROUP X TIME	2.21	1,30	2.21	0.62	ns

Figure 6.52 (6.6.4.5)   Factor 6 Physical and Gross-Motor

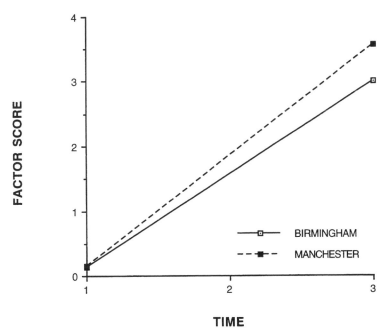

TIME

	TIME 1	TIME 2	TIME 3
BIRMINGHAM			
N	18		18
MEAN	0.14		3.00
SD	4.28		5.45
MANCHESTER			
N	17		15
MEAN	0.16		3.58
SD	5.68		6.75

SOURCE OF VARIATION	SUM OF SQUARES	df	Var. Est.	F	Sig.
GROUP	0.31	1,30	0.31	0.01	ns
TIME	239.68	1,30	239.68	114.81	<0.001
GROUP X TIME	1.45	1,30	1.45	0.69	ns

Figure 6.53 (6.6.4.6)   Factor 8 Behaviour Problems

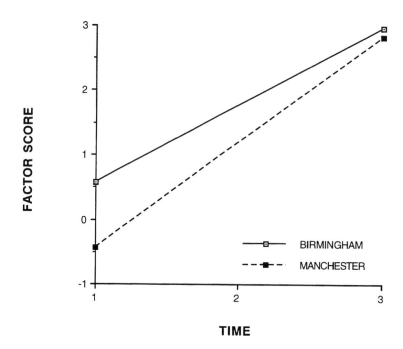

	TIME 1	TIME 2	TIME 3
BIRMINGHAM			
N	18		18
MEAN	0.58		2.96
SD	3.22		3.89
MANCHESTER			
N	17		15
MEAN	-0.44		2.83
SD	3.55		4.33

SOURCE OF VARIATION	SUM OF SQUARES	df	Var. Est.	F	Sig.
GROUP	11.48	1,30	11.48	0.42	ns
TIME	155.11	1,30	155.11	147.56	<0.001
GROUP X TIME	2.18	1,30	2.18	2.07	ns

Figure 6.54 (6.6.4.7)   Factor 10 Independence and Social

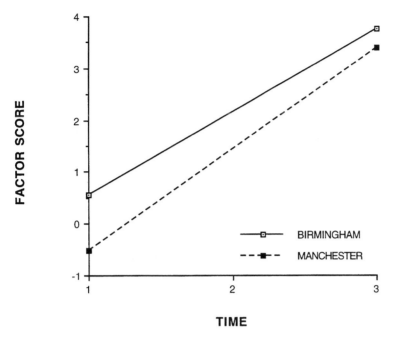

TIME

	TIME 1	TIME 2	TIME 3
BIRMINGHAM			
N	18		18
MEAN	0.57		3.77
SD	3.20		3.90
MANCHESTER			
N	17		15
MEAN	-0.50		3.40
SD	3.74		4.28

SOURCE OF VARIATION	SUM OF SQUARES	df	Var. Est.	F	Sig.
GROUP	14.36	1,30	14.36	0.51	ns
TIME	235.77	1,30	235.77	197.21	<0.001
GROUP X TIME	2.04	1,30	2.04	1.70	ns

221

Figure 6.55 (6.2.2.1)   Developmental Profile II: Academic (Parent Report)

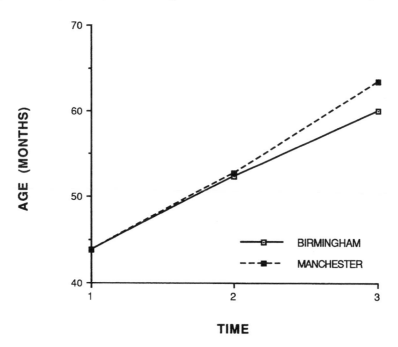

	TIME 1	TIME 2	TIME 3
BIRMINGHAM			
N	18	19	19
MEAN	43.8	52.3	60.0
SD	13.8	12.7	16.0
MANCHESTER			
N	17	17	17
MEAN	43.8	52.7	63.4
SD	14.3	17.2	19.9

SOURCE OF VARIATION	SUM OF SQUARES	df	Var. Est.	F	Sig.
GROUP	36.64	1,33	36.64	0.05	ns
TIME	5624.69	2,66	2812.34	64.00	<0.001
GROUP X TIME	56.50	2,66	28.25	0.64	ns

TIME 1 vs TIME 2, t=-6.16, df=34, p<0.001;
TIME 2 vs TIME 3, t=-6.89, df=35, p<0.001.

Figure 6.56 (6.2.2.1)　Developmental Profile II: Intelligence Quotient (Parent Report)

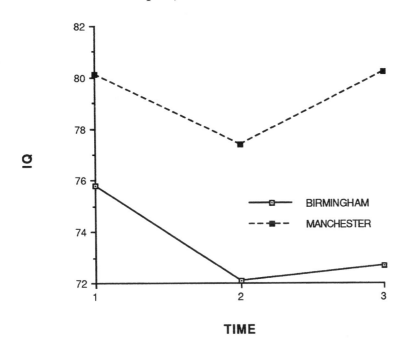

TIME

	TIME 1	TIME 2	TIME 3
BIRMINGHAM			
N	18	19	19
MEAN	75.8	72.1	71.7
SD	21.6	17.9	19.6
MANCHESTER			
N	17	17	17
MEAN	80.1	77.4	80.2
SD	25.8	24.3	25.8

SOURCE OF VARIATION	SUM OF SQUARES	df	Var. Est.	F	Sig.
GROUP	867.68	1,33	867.68	0.63	ns
TIME	166.99	2,66	83.49	0.97	ns
GROUP X TIME	72.59	2,66	36.29	0.42	ns

TIME 1 vs TIME 2, t=1.43, df=34, ns;
TIME 2 vs TIME 3, t=-0.68, df=35, ns.

Figure 6.57 (6.2.2.2)   Developmental Profile II: Communication (Parent Report)

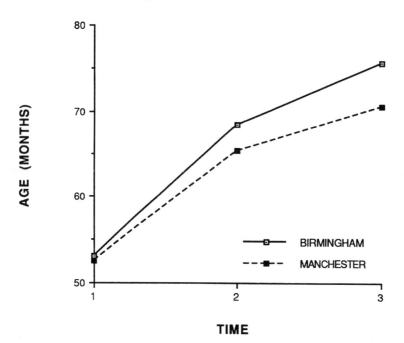

	TIME 1	TIME 2	TIME 3
BIRMINGHAM			
N	18	19	19
MEAN	53.1	68.4	75.7
SD	17.4	17.3	23.1
MANCHESTER			
N	17	17	17
MEAN	52.5	65.4	70.6
SD	20.1	24.2	23.2

SOURCE OF VARIATION	SUM OF SQUARES	df	Var. Est.	F	Sig.
GROUP	228.91	1,33	228.91	0.19	ns
TIME	7562.43	2,66	3781.21	63.23	<0.001
GROUP X TIME	79.91	2,66	39.96	0.67	ns

TIME 1 vs TIME 2, t=-8.86, df=34, p<0.001;
TIME 2 vs TIME 3, t=-3.60, df=35, p<0.01.

Figure 6.58 (6.2.2.3) Developmental Profile II: Physical (Parent Report)

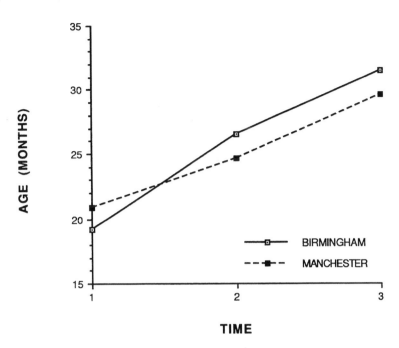

	TIME 1	TIME 2	TIME 3
BIRMINGHAM			
N	18	19	19
MEAN	19.2	26.5	31.5
SD	10.3	13.1	18.7
MANCHESTER			
N	17	17	17
MEAN	20.9	24.7	29.6
SD	9.5	11.4	16.2

SOURCE OF VARIATION	SUM OF SQUARES	df	Var. Est.	F	Sig.
GROUP	37.66	1,33	37.66	0.08	ns
TIME	2105.70	2,66	1052.85	26.89	<0.001
GROUP X TIME	111.95	2,66	55.97	1.43	ns

TIME 1 vs TIME 2, t=-4.88, df= 34, p<0.001;
TIME 2 vs TIME 3, t=-3.48, df=35, p<0.01.

Figure 6.59 (6.2.2.4)　Developmental Profile II: Social (Parent Report)

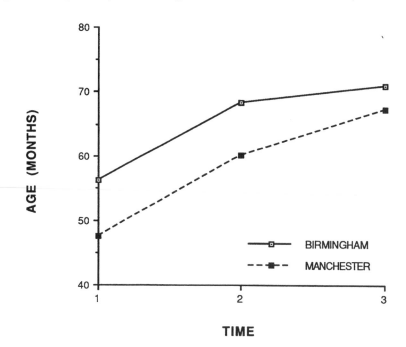

	TIME 1	TIME 2	TIME 3
BIRMINGHAM			
N	18	19	19
MEAN	56.3	68.3	70.9
SD	12.4	13.0	17.2
MANCHESTER			
N	17	17	17
MEAN	47.5	60.2	67.3
SD	15.4	15.6	17.4

SOURCE OF VARIATION	SUM OF SQUARES	df	Var. Est.	F	Sig.
GROUP	1251.03	1,33	1251.03	2.12	ns
TIME	5519.19	2,66	2759.59	45.05	<0.001
GROUP X TIME	135.87	2,66	67.94	1.11	ns

TIME 1 vs TIME 2, t=-7.52, df=34, p<0.001;
TIME 2 vs TIME 3, t=-2.67, df=35, p<0.05.

Figure 6.60 (6.2.2.5) Developmental Profile II: Self-Help (Parent Report)

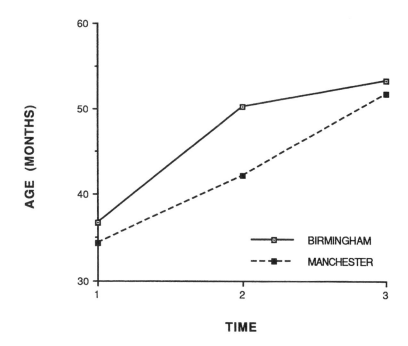

	TIME 1	TIME 2	TIME 3
BIRMINGHAM			
N	18	19	19
MEAN	36.7	50.2	53.3
SD	16.0	18.2	25.3
MANCHESTER			
N	17	17	17
MEAN	34.4	42.2	51.8
SD	12.2	18.3	23.4

SOURCE OF VARIATION	SUM OF SQUARES	df	Var. Est.	F	Sig.
GROUP	587.85	1,33	587.85	0.63	ns
TIME	5562.71	2,66	2781.35	27.60	<0.001
GROUP X TIME	263.20	2,66	131.60	1.31	ns

TIME 1 vs TIME 2, t=-5.56, df=34, p<0.001;
TIME 2 vs TIME 3, t=-2.84, df=35, p<0.01.

Figure 6.61 (6.2.3.1) Pictorial Test of Intelligence: Immediate Recall (Direct Test)

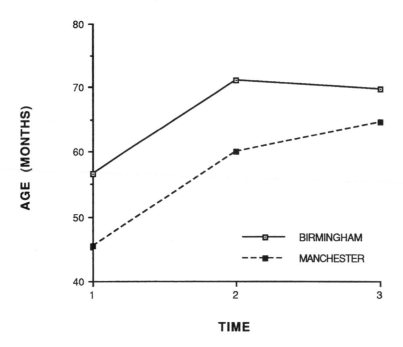

	TIME 1	TIME 2	TIME 3
BIRMINGHAM			
N	19	19	19
MEAN	56.5	71.1	69.8
SD	22.1	20.7	21.8
MANCHESTER			
N	17	17	17
MEAN	45.4	60.0	64.6
SD	20.8	25.0	25.1

SOURCE OF VARIATION	SUM OF SQUARES	df	Var. Est.	F	Sig.
GROUP	2249.80	1,34	2249.80	1.99	ns
TIME	5737.11	2,68	2868.56	14.27	<0.001
GROUP X TIME	209.11	2,68	104.56	0.52	ns

TIME 1 vs TIME 2, t=-4.06, df=35, p<0.001;
TIME 2 vs TIME 3, t=-0.58, df=35, ns.

Figure 6.62 (6.2.3.2) Pictorial Test of Intelligence: Form Discrimination
(Direct Test)

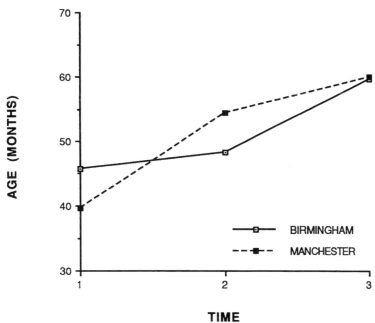

	TIME 1	TIME 2	TIME 3
BIRMINGHAM			
N	19	19	19
MEAN	45.8	48.3	59.8
SD	11.9	15.2	24.3
MANCHESTER			
N	17	17	17
MEAN	39.5	54.4	60.0
SD	15.0	26.3	27.2

SOURCE OF VARIATION	SUM OF SQUARES	df	Var. Est.	F	Sig.
GROUP	0.01	1,34	0.01	0.00	ns
TIME	5346.83	2,68	2673.42	18.21	<0.001
GROUP X TIME	678.83	2,68	339.42	2.31	ns

TIME 1 vs TIME 2, t=-2.63, df=35, p<0.05;
TIME 2 vs TIME 3, t=-3.36, df=35, p<0.01.

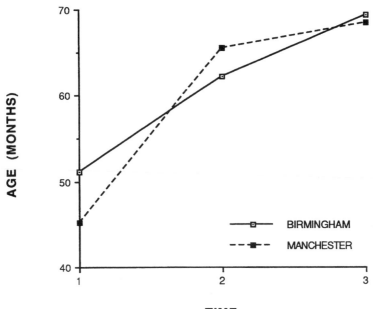

TIME

	TIME 1	TIME 2	TIME 3
BIRMINGHAM			
N	19	19	19
MEAN	51.2	62.2	69.3
SD	12.1	18.0	23.3
MANCHESTER			
N	17	17	17
MEAN	45.2	65.5	68.5
SD	11.8	22.1	25.4

SOURCE OF VARIATION	SUM OF SQUARES	df	Var. Est.	F	Sig.
GROUP	38.04	1,34	38.04	0.05	ns
TIME	8383.06	2,68	4191.53	23.45	<0.001
GROUP X TIME	384.73	2,68	192.36	1.08	ns

TIME 1 vs TIME 2, t=-4.73, df=35, p<0.001;
TIME 2 vs TIME 3, t=-1.76, df=35, ns.

Figure 6.64 (6.2.3.4) Pictorial Test of Intelligence: Information and Comprehension (Direct Test)

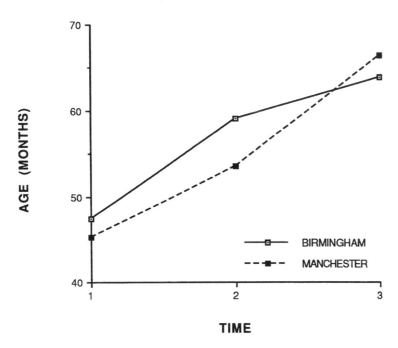

	TIME 1	TIME 2	TIME 3
BIRMINGHAM			
N	19	19	19
MEAN	47.4	59.1	63.8
SD	12.8	13.6	17.7
MANCHESTER			
N	17	17	17
MEAN	45.2	53.6	66.4
SD	12.0	14.8	25.3

SOURCE OF VARIATION	SUM OF SQUARES	df	Var. Est.	F	Sig.
GROUP	75.79	1,34	75.79	0.13	ns
TIME	6352.45	2,68	3176.22	24.73	<0.001
GROUP X TIME	288.45	2,68	144.22	1.12	ns

TIME 1 vs TIME 2, t=-4.12, df=35, p<0.001;
TIME 2 vs TIME 3, t=-3.37, df=35, p<0.01.

Figure 6.65 (6.2.3.5) Pictorial Test of Intelligence: Size and Number (Direct Test)

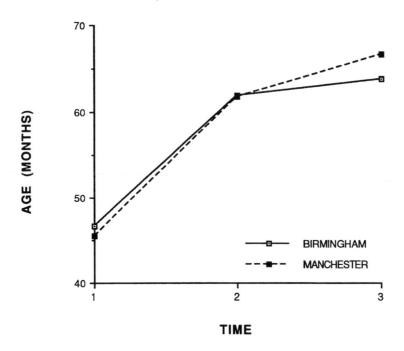

	TIME 1	TIME 2	TIME 3
BIRMINGHAM			
N	19	19	19
MEAN	46.7	61.9	63.8
SD	10.3	13.9	16.3
MANCHESTER			
N	17	17	17
MEAN	45.5	61.8	66.7
SD	13.6	19.1	20.2

SOURCE OF VARIATION	SUM OF SQUARES	df	Var. Est.	F	Sig.
GROUP	7.46	1,34	7.46	0.01	ns
TIME	7458.09	2,68	3729.04	38.59	<0.001
GROUP X TIME	82.09	2,68	41.04	0.42	ns

TIME 1 vs TIME 2, t=-7.02, df=35, p<0.001;
TIME 2 vs TIME 3, t=-1.47, df=35, ns.

Figure 6.66 (6.2.3.6)   Pictorial Test of Intelligence: Picture Vocabulary
(Direct Test)

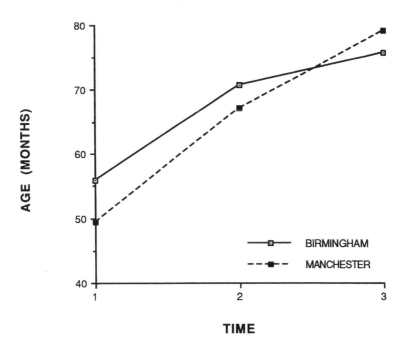

	TIME 1	TIME 2	TIME 3
BIRMINGHAM			
N	19	19	19
MEAN	55.9	70.7	75.8
SD	21.2	19.2	19.5
MANCHESTER			
N	17	17	17
MEAN	49.4	67.2	79.2
SD	18.6	21.5	28.6

SOURCE OF VARIATION	SUM OF SQUARES	df	Var. Est.	F	Sig.
GROUP	127.87	1,34	127.87	0.13	ns
TIME	11453.77	2,68	5726.88	28.89	<0.001
GROUP X TIME	465.77	2,68	232.88	1.17	ns

TIME 1 vs TIME 2, t=-4.98, df=35, p<0.001;
TIME 2 vs TIME 3, t=-2.22, df=35, p<0.05.

Figure 6.67 (6.2.3.7)   Pictorial Test of Intelligence: General Cognition
(Direct Test)

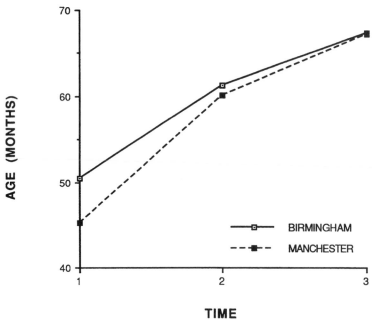

TIME

	TIME 1	TIME 2	TIME 3
BIRMINGHAM			
N	19	19	19
MEAN	50.5	61.3	67.3
SD	10.0	11.8	16.1
MANCHESTER			
N	17	17	17
MEAN	45.3	60.1	67.2
SD	13.5	16.6	21.9

SOURCE OF VARIATION	SUM OF SQUARES	df	Var. Est.	F	Sig.
GROUP	124.98	1,34	124.98	0.20	ns
TIME	6962.47	2,68	3481.23	87.58	<0.001
GROUP X TIME	129.91	2,68	64.96	1.63	ns

TIME 1 vs TIME 2, t=-8.74, df=35, p<0.001;
TIME 2 vs TIME 3, t=-5.49, df=35, p<0.001.

234

Figure 6.68 (6.2.3.7)   Pictorial Test of Intelligence: Intelligence Quotient
(Direct Test)

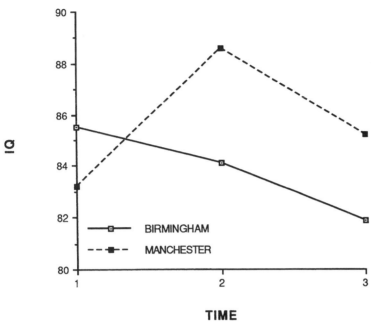

TIME

	TIME 1	TIME 2	TIME 3
BIRMINGHAM			
N	19	19	19
MEAN	85.5	84.1	81.9
SD	20.0	18.4	21.9
MANCHESTER			
N	17	17	17
MEAN	83.2	88.6	85.2
SD	25.1	27.4	29.3

SOURCE OF VARIATION	SUM OF SQUARES	df	Var. Est.	F	Sig.
GROUP	91.34	1,34	94.34	0.06	ns
TIME	154.31	2,68	77.15	1.63	ns
GROUP X TIME	237.72	2,68	118.86	2.51	ns

TIME 1 vs TIME 2, t=-0.95, df=35, ns;
TIME 2 vs TIME 3, t=2.38, df=35, p<0.05.

Figure 6.69 (6.2.5.3) Articulation (Direct Test)

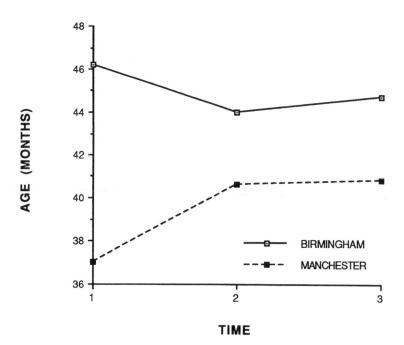

	TIME 1	TIME 2	TIME 3
BIRMINGHAM			
N	18	19	19
MEAN	46.2	44.0	44.7
SD	12.7	10.7	10.9
MANCHESTER			
N	17	17	17
MEAN	37.0	40.6	40.8
SD	3.0	10.0	9.0

SOURCE OF VARIATION	SUM OF SQUARES	df	Var. Est.	F	Sig.
GROUP	890.33	1,33	890.33	3.46	ns
TIME	34.09	2,66	17.05	0.85	ns
GROUP X TIME	150.06	2,66	75.03	3.72	<0.05

TIME 1 vs TIME 2, t=-0.63, df=34, ns;
TIME 2 vs TIME 3, t=-0.81, df=35, ns.

236

Figure 6.70 (6.2.5.4) Expressive Verbal (Direct Test)

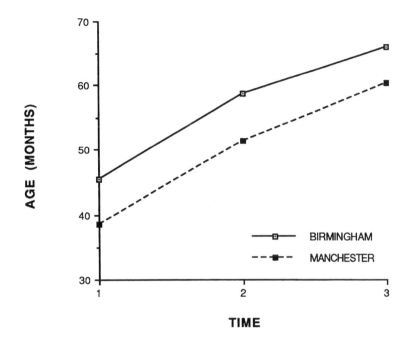

	TIME 1	TIME 2	TIME 3
BIRMINGHAM			
N	18	19	19
MEAN	45.3	58.7	66.1
SD	19.1	22.2	22.6
MANCHESTER			
N	17	17	17
MEAN	38.5	51.3	60.5
SD	15.0	19.5	22.3

SOURCE OF VARIATION	SUM OF SQUARES	df	Var. Est.	F	Sig.
GROUP	1199.87	1,33	1199.87	1.11	ns
TIME	8256.67	2,66	4128.34	44.45	<0.001
GROUP X TIME	15.36	2,66	7.68	0.08	ns

TIME 1 vs TIME 2, t=-5.51, df=34, p<0.001;
TIME 2 vs TIME 3, t=-4.36, df=35, p<0.001.

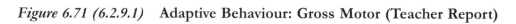

Figure 6.71 (6.2.9.1) Adaptive Behaviour: Gross Motor (Teacher Report)

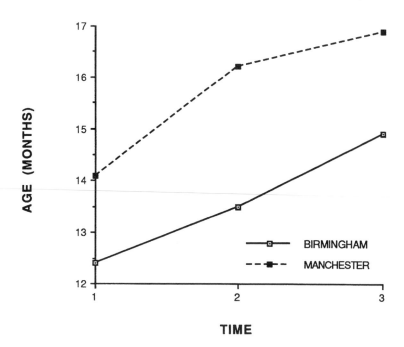

	TIME 1	TIME 2	TIME 3
BIRMINGHAM			
N	19	19	19
MEAN	12.4	13.5	14.9
SD	5.3	6.2	7.5
MANCHESTER			
N	17	17	17
MEAN	14.1	16.2	16.9
SD	7.7	12.4	15.9

SOURCE OF VARIATION	SUM OF SQUARES	df	Var. Est.	F	Sig.
GROUP	122.00	1,34	122.00	0.48	ns
TIME	127.54	2,68	63.77	4.27	<0.05
GROUP X TIME	3.91	2,68	1.96	0.13	ns

TIME 1 vs TIME 2, t=-2.04, df=35, p<0.05;
TIME 2 vs TIME 3, t=-1.59, df=35, ns.

238

Figure 6.72 (6.2.9.2) Adaptive Behaviour: Interpersonal (Teacher Report)

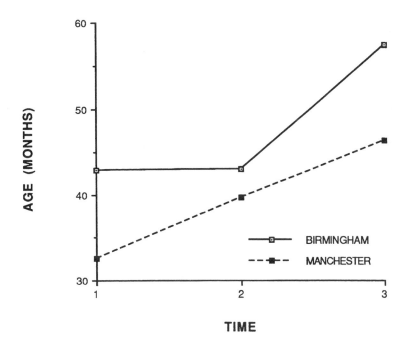

	TIME 1	TIME 2	TIME 3
BIRMINGHAM			
N	19	19	19
MEAN	43.0	43.1	57.5
SD	31.2	37.7	33.9
MANCHESTER			
N	17	17	17
MEAN	32.5	39.8	46.4
SD	28.8	21.7	27.9

SOURCE OF VARIATION	SUM OF SQUARES	df	Var. Est.	F	Sig.
GROUP	1850.28	1,34	1850.28	0.85	ns
TIME	3914.42	2,68	1957.21	5.76	<0.01
GROUP X TIME	346.38	2,68	173.19	0.51	ns

TIME 1 vs TIME 2, t=-0.94, df=35, ns;
TIME 2 vs TIME 3, t=-2.25, df=35, p<0.05.

Figure 6.73 (6.2.9.3) Adaptive Behaviour: Play (Teacher Report)

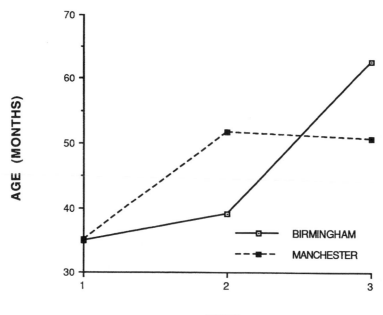

	TIME 1	TIME 2	TIME 3
BIRMINGHAM			
N	19	19	19
MEAN	34.9	39.1	62.6
SD	19.7	19.4	32.9
MANCHESTER			
N	17	17	17
MEAN	35.1	51.7	50.7
SD	22.7	22.1	24.1

SOURCE OF VARIATION	SUM OF SQUARES	df	Var. Est.	F	Sig.
GROUP	2.41	1,34	2.41	0.00	ns
TIME	8405.58	2,68	4202.79	14.92	<0.001
GROUP X TIME	2710.39	2,68	1355.20	4.81	<0.05

TIME 1 vs TIME 2, t=-3.43, df=35, p<0.01;
TIME 2 vs TIME 3, t=-2.45, df=35, p<0.05.

Figure 6.74 (6.2.9.4)   Adaptive Behaviour: Activities of Daily Living (Teacher Report)

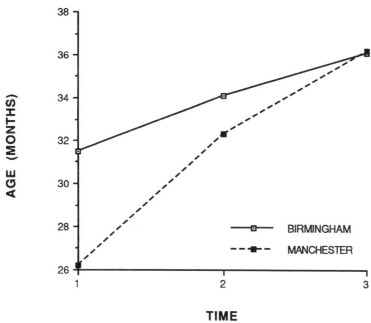

TIME

	TIME 1	TIME 2	TIME 3
BIRMINGHAM			
N	19	19	19
MEAN	31.5	34.1	36.1
SD	11.9	14.1	12.4
MANCHESTER			
N	17	17	17
MEAN	26.2	32.3	36.2
SD	8.3	10.6	13.9

SOURCE OF VARIATION	SUM OF SQUARES	df	Var. Est.	F	Sig.
GROUP	145.38	1,34	145.38	0.38	ns
TIME	946.38	2,68	482.19	16.93	<0.001
GROUP X TIME	135.38	2,68	67.69	2.38	ns

TIME 1 vs TIME 2, t=-4.77, df=35, p<0.001;
TIME 2 vs TIME 3, t=-2.24, df=35, p<0.05.

Appendix 6.1

Letter sent to local education and local health authorities seeking cooperation in the research project

Dear . . . .,

We are seeking your cooperation in a research project aimed at evaluating Conductive Education (CE). This system of teaching the motor disordered, pioneered in Hungary, is being brought to the United Kingdom. The András Pető Institute in Budapest is collaborating with the Foundation for Conductive Education in Birmingham in setting up a duplicate of the Hungarian system. Work underway includes the conversion of a former school in Birmingham to provide facilities the same as those in the Hungarian Institute. The Hungarians have selected and trained a group of British teachers to become 'conductors'. They have also selected a sample of British pupils whom they think will benefit from CE, and are supervising the trainee conductors as they teach these pupils. The first intake are children aged between three and four years with cerebral palsy.

The Department of Education and Science has given funds to evaluate CE as established in Birmingham. The research is being carried out from the Department of Psychology, University of Birmingham, independently from the Birmingham Institute of Conductive Education but with the Institute's cooperation. The research has four objectives:

1.   to determine the extent to which the form of CE developed in Birmingham is an accurate replica of that established at the Pető Institute.

2.   to make explicit the principles upon which CE operates, and which may be crucial to its success.

3.   to show whether CE produces a pattern of improvement in the social, mental and motor development of cerebral palsied children, which differs from that found in existing British programmes.

4.   to define the limits of applicability of CE in Britain.

We are seeking groups of children in existing British programmes who would be suitable to compare against the children in CE. The Department of Education and Science has established a Steering Committee to monitor and advise on the research. The Committee has put forward the name of your (Education/Health) Authority as being a possible source of comparison children.

We need children with cerebral palsy who are not necessarily matched initially to those in CE, but who are enrolled in reputable British programmes. We intend to measure the progress of all children in domains specified by the objectives of the programmes being compared. The purpose is to show that children achieve different rates of improvement in motor, mental and social domains, in line with specific sets of objectives. The nomination of your authority is a sign of the high opinion held of the provisions made for children with cerebral palsy.

We would welcome the opportunity to discuss with you the research, and whether you would in principle be willing to put forward the names of Institutes and children to serve as comparison groups in this evaluation.

Yours sincerely,

Appendix 6.2

Letter sent to parents of potential comparison children seeking their cooperation in the evaluation.

Dear . . . .,

The Department of Education and Science has commissioned the University of Birmingham to carry out an evaluation of different programmes of education for cerebral palsied children. One programme is conductive education at the Birmingham Institute of Conductive Education. (Local authority) has been selected as a comparison, because programmes being offered are highly regarded and are believed to compare favourably with the Birmingham programme. The aim is to show whether different programmes of education achieve good results in different areas of children's development.

We would like the opportunity to assess whether your child could be included in the (Local authority) group. The selection procedure, involving the assessment of basic functional abilities, would be carried out by a team from the University of Birmingham who will travel to (local authority) in (date).

If your child is selected for the study, there will be no disruption to the programme of education. Rather, what has been planned in (Local authority) will be carried out normally. The only difference will be that your child's development will be followed, perhaps more comprehensively than usual, over the next three years. This will involve directly assessing your child from time to time at school, as well as asking you and the teachers about your child's progress. All this work will be carried out in (local authority).

There will also be a requirement for your child to attend the Orthotic Locomotor Assessment Unit at Oswestry once a year for a physical examination and an assessment of walking. We would like each child to be accompanied by a parent on this occasion. The visit will be arranged by the team from Birmingham at no cost to yourself.

All results and all information gathered in the study will be treated in the strictest of confidence, and individual children will not be identified in any reports. On the other hand, there will be ample opportunity for you to meet the team carrying out the study to obtain more information and to discuss results.

We hope you will agree to your child's participation in this study. The results will show how well children progress in their different programmes of education, and will be beneficial in the design of new programmes. We would be grateful if you could kindly return the accompanying slip in the reply-paid envelope supplied.

Yours sincerely,

Appendix 6.3

Correlations between raw scores and chronological age at testing, based on Time 1 data from children in the Birmingham and Manchester groups.

Developmental Profile II.   Academic (0.25), Communication (0.25), Physical (0.05), Social (0.03), Self-Help (0.35).

Pictorial Test of Intelligence.   General Cognition (0.23).

Language Assessment.   Motor Control 1 (0.23), Motor Control 2 (0.06), Motor Control 3 (0.15), Receptive Non-Verbal (0.28), Expressive Non-Verbal (0.17), Receptive verbal (0.27), Articulation (0.40), Expressive Verbal (0.19).

Fine-Motor Independence.   Independence (0.11), Object Transfer 1 (−0.08), Object Transfer 2 (−0.11), Manipulation (−0.14), Two-Hand Coordination (0.01), Pen Placement (0.26), Drawing (0.30).

Gross-Motor Assessment.   Postural Independence (0.12), Position Changing Independence (0.00), Crawling Independence (−0.02), Walking Independence (−0.10), Preferred Locomotion Independence (0.20), Position Changing (0.01), Crawling (−0.07), Walking (−0.06), Preferred Locomotion (−0.07).

Adaptive Behaviour.   Gross-Motor (−0.19), Interpersonal (0.90), Play (−0.10), Activities of Daily Living (0.09), Attention and Control (−0.24).

Behaviour Problems   (0.25).

Appendix 6.4

Functional and physical variables used in a principal-components analysis of Time 1 assessment data from children in the Birmingham and Manchester groups.

Developmental Profile II: Academic (Section 6.2.2.1)
Developmental Profile II: Communication (Section 6.2.2.2)
Developmental Profile II: Physical (Section 6.2.2.3)
Developmental Profile II: Social (Section 6.2.2.4)
Developmental Profile II: Self-Help (Section 6.2.2.5)

Pictorial Test of Intelligence: General Cognition (Section 6.2.3.7)

Language: Motor Control 1 (Section 6.2.5.1.1)
Language: Motor Control 2 (Section 6.2.5.1.2)
Language: Motor Control 3 (Section 6.2.5.2.1)
Language: Receptive Non-Verbal (Section 6.2.5.2.2)
Language: Expressive Non-Verbal (Section 6.2.5.2.3)
Language: Receptive Verbal (Section 6.2.5.2.4)
Language: Articulation (Section 6.2.5.3)
Language: Expressive Verbal (Section 6.2.5.4)

Fine-Motor: Independence (Section 6.2.6.1)
Fine-Motor: Object Transfer 1 (Section 6.2.6.2)
Fine-Motor: Object Transfer 2 (Section 6.2.6.3)
Fine-Motor: Manipulation (Section 6.2.6.4)
Fine-Motor: Two-Hand Coordination (Section 6.2.6.5)
Fine-Motor: Pen Placement (Section 6.2.6.6)
Fine-Motor: Drawing (Section 6.2.6.7)

Gross-Motor: Postural Independence (Section 6.2.7.1)
Gross-Motor: Position Changing Independence (Section 6.2.7.2)
Gross-Motor: Crawling Independence (Section 6.2.7.3)
Gross-Motor: Walking Independence (Section 6.2.7.4)
Gross-Motor: Preferred Locomotion Independence (Section 6.2.7.5)
Gross-Motor: Position Changing (Section 6.2.7.7)
Gross-Motor: Crawling (Section 6.2.7.8)
Gross-Motor: Walking (Section 6.2.7.9)
Gross-Motor: Preferred Locomotion (Section 6.2.7.10)

Physical: Hip Mobility (Section 6.2.8.1)
Physical: Hamstring Extensibility (Section 6.2.8.2)
Physical: Height (Section 6.2.8.3)
Physical: Weight (Section 6.2.8.4)
Physical: Neurology (Section 6.2.8.5)

Adaptive Behaviour: Gross-Motor (Section 6.2.9.1)
Adaptive Behaviour: Interpersonal (Section 6.2.9.2)
Adaptive Behaviour: Play (Section 6.2.9.3)
Adaptive Behaviour: Activities of Daily Living (Section 6.2.9.4)
Adaptive Behaviour: Attention and Control (Section 6.2.9.5)

Behaviour Problems: (Section 6.2.10)

Appendix 6.5

Malaise Inventory completed as a questionnaire by mothers.

YOUR HEALTH:

Please tick **one** box for **each** of the following questions

		YES	NO
1)	Do you often have backache?	☐	☐
2)	Do you feel tired most of the time?	☐	☐
3)	Do you often feel miserable or depressed?	☐	☐
4)	Do you often have bad headaches?	☐	☐
5)	Do you often get worried about things?	☐	☐
6)	Do you usually have great difficulty in falling asleep or staying asleep?	☐	☐
7)	Do you usually wake unnecessarily early in the morning?	☐	☐
8)	Do you wear yourself out worrying about your health?	☐	☐
9)	Do you often get into a violent rage?	☐	☐
10)	Do people often annoy and irritate you?	☐	☐
11)	Have you at times had a twitching of the face, head or shoulders?	☐	☐
12)	Do you often suddenly become scared for no good reason?	☐	☐
13)	Are you scared to be alone when there are no friends near you?	☐	☐
14)	Are you easily upset or irritated?	☐	☐
15)	Are you frightened of going out alone or of meeting people?	☐	☐
16)	Are you constantly keyed up and jittery?	☐	☐
17)	Do you suffer from indigestion?	☐	☐
18)	Do you often suffer from an upset stomach?	☐	☐
19)	Is your appetite poor?	☐	☐
20)	Does every little thing get on your nerves and wear you out?	☐	☐

21)	Does your heart often race like mad?	☐	☐
22)	Do you often have bad pains in your eyes?	☐	☐
23)	Are you troubled with rheumatism or fibrositis?	☐	☐
24)	Have you ever had a nervous breakdown?	☐	☐

Appendix 6.6

Attitude questionnaire completed by mothers.

Here is a picture of a ladder. At the bottom of the ladder is the worst life you might reasonably expect to have. At the top is the best life you might expect to have. The other rungs are in between. WRITE A NUMBER ON THE LINE TO THE LEFT OF EACH QUESTION BELOW.

9	Best I could expect to have
8	
7	
6	
5	
4	
3	
2	
1	Worst I could expect to have

1. Where on the ladder would best describe how you feel about your **life as a whole** . . . on which rung would you put it?

2. Where on the ladder would you put **the help** your child is receiving . . . on which rung?

3. Where on the ladder would you put **the progress** your child is making . . . on which rung would you put it?

Appendix 6.7

Function of the children assessed by the research team, grouped under seven headings.

---

1. Mental Functioning

Categories of Function	Types of Items
Visual short-term memory	Memory of visual patterns, search for something just hidden.
Visual matching, discrimination	Match forms, discriminate shapes.
Concept formation	Categorisation, generalisation.
General knowledge	General understanding, use of objects, properties of objects, origin of things.
Premaths, maths	Size, measurement, number concept, number symbol, counting, arithmetic operators, money, purchasing including change.
Time concept	Telling time, days of week, activity/time association.
Colour naming	
Pre-reading, reading	Visual sequential memory, letter recognition, printed word recognition, comprehension of printed word, grammar, reading, meaning of words, memory of telephone numbers or addresses.

---

2. Communication

Categories of Function	Types of Items
Non-verbal comprehension	Understanding gestures, non-verbal imitation, task imitation, knowledge of other's emotions or feelings, respond to hints or cues.
Non-verbal communication	Use of gestures, waving, hugging, letter writing, poem/song writing, positive or negative reactions, use of symbols or signs, facial gestures, sharing attention, attention seeking.
Verbal comprehension	Understanding spoken words, picture/word association, object/word association, carry

out commands, follow radio programme, retell plot, recall story content.

Muscle control	Control of facial muscles and speech apparatus with or without sound, drooling, winking, whistle, vocal noise play, lips, tongue, palate, jaw.
Articulation of consonants	
Verbal expression	Babble talk, size words, counting, days of week, sound/word imitation, word/object association, sentences, repeat rhyme, rhyming words, word/picture association, singe rhyme, tell story from picture, telephone conversation, sing a song, tell story without picture, use argument, read aloud, retell plot, phrase imitation, name associated with familiar person, recite poems.

3. Fine Motor Functioning

Categories of Function	Types of Items
Grasping, placing, releasing objects	Objects of various shapes, various sizes, various weights, constrained, unconstrained.
Differentiated control of fingers	Finger thumb opposition, manipulation, unwrapping, cutting out, key, door latches.
Two-hand coordination	
Use of pencil and paper	Marking, copying, drawing, colouring.
Writing	Letters, words, printing, script.
Throwing, catching	

4. Gross Motor Functioning

Categories of Function	Types of Items
Control of static posture	Lying, sitting, kneeling, standing.
Position changing	Lying-sitting, sitting-kneeling, kneeling-standing, sitting-standing, standing-sitting, rolling.
Crawling, creeping	
Walking without aids	Walking, carrying, avoiding objects, running.
Stairs, climbing	Up, down, holding, not holding.
Jumping, hopping, skipping	Up and down, forward, rope, hopscotch.

Bicycle, tricycle

Rollerskates, skateboard, iceskate

Sports

5. Personal Behaviour

Categories of Function	Types of Items
Sense of identity	Concept of 'my', jealousy, own sex, own body, own emotions, likes/dislikes, preferences, self recognition, own address, own age.
Solitary activities	Play, occupy, hobby, build/mend, use of TV for enjoyment or information.
Manners, socially acceptable behaviour	
Secrets	Keeping secrets.
Make believe	Something is not real (eg., santa claus), using real objects in imaginative play, pretend.
Attention span, self control	Listen in groups, application to task without supervision, concentrate with distractions, quieten down.
Behaviour problems	Thumb/finger sucking, sleeping, nail biting, tics/twitches, crying, teeth grinding, temper tantrums, rocking, self-injury.

6. Interpersonal Behaviour

Categories of Function	Types of Items
Imitation	Actions, words, phrases, tasks.
Interest in others	Childrens activities, other's sex, other's names, ownership by others, family relationship (eg., uncle, cousin).
Responsiveness to others	Wants attention, negative responsiveness, positive responsiveness, awareness of other's emotions, responding to instructions, preference for some others, application to task with supervision, overcome withdrawal from others.
Pleasing others	Handle something breakable, respond to other's good fortune, initiating topic of

	interest to others, gifts for others, other's anniversaries, helping.
Games	Rule following, sharing, turn taking, play/game with one other, play/game in group, interaction games, activities with others.
Friendship	Particular friends, best friend, group of friends, visiting friends.
Attending groups or clubs	Exploring new places, school or non-school sports or events.

7. Self-Help Behaviour

Categories of Function	Types of Items
Drinking	Sucking, bottle, straw, cup, glass.
Eating	Solid foods, chewing, use of spoon/fork/knife, understanding edible/non-edible.
Dressing, undressing	Helping, doing, clothing, footwear, buttons, laces, zippers, fasteners, changing clothes, choosing clothes.
Toileting	Indicating soiled pants, indicating need (toilet training), use of potty, use of WC, use of paper.
Washing, drying	Hands, face, body, use of bath, use of shower, tooth wash.
Grooming	Brush hair, comb hair, clean/cut fingernails.
Health	Wipe nose, care for nose, cover mouth when coughing, avoiding contagion, care for cuts/burns, take medicine, thermometer, contact doctor.
Preparing food	Bowl of cereal, sandwich, eggs, canned food, cooking
Responsibility and chores	Helping, carrying out tasks independently, putting away toys, sole care of animal.
Getting about	At home unsupervised, understanding dangers (stairs, glass, busy street, animals), answering telephone, using telephone, managing money, purchasing, use of radio or TV for information or news, remembering telephone numbers and addresses, visiting neighbour.

Appendix 6.8

Developmental Background Interview Schedule

1. Purpose of interview with parents: explore understanding.

2. Family composition.

3. Think back over year, recall landmarks; any records kept?

4. Consider each heading on Data sheet: were there any events or changes which affected . . . .'s progress over this period? For example, input from family, from other professionals or helpers, medical intervention or treatment, family changes etc?

5. What difference do you think this/these changes made to . . . .?
   (Take each one in turn, note effect on any of these functions).

   COGNITION
   COMMUNICATION
   FINE-MOTOR
   GROSS-MOTOR
   PERSONAL
   INTERPERSONAL
   SELF-HELP

6. Describe the usual pattern of activity in the family between . . . .'s homecoming and bedtime.

   What sort of activities go on in the family at weekends? In the holidays?

Appendix 6.9

Developmental Background Interview: Data Sheet.

Child: Date:

Respondent:

Notes:

INTERVIEW DATA

CHILD'S NAME . . . . DATE . . . .

Areas of Function	INPUT 1 Family Input & Effect		INPUT 2 Other Input eg., Speech Physio-therapy Teaching		INPUT 3 Medical or Surgical Input		INPUT 4 Other Input eg., Club Family Problem Illness	
Cognition								
Communication								
Fine-motor								
Gross-motor								
Personal								
Interpersonal								
Self-help								

[+=helped   x=hindered   o=outcome uncertain]

Appendix 6.10

Letter sent to Birmingham families

24th August 1990.

Dear . . . .,

As you know, the research project on Conductive Education is studying the progress of all the children who have attended the Institute and a comparison group of children in Manchester. As part of this study, we need to know about anything which has been happening which may have a bearing on the children's development. It is fairly common, for example, for children in all types of education to have help out of school. On the other hand, prolonged illness or surgery can hold a child back. It is important for us to know about these things if we are to understand how a child is progressing.

To help with this part of the study, Jeanne Downton has recently joined the research team. She has a lot of experience of working with children and families, and would like to talk with all the parents of children who have attended the Institute. She will also later be seeing the parents of the comparison children in Manchester.

Jeanne would therefore like some time to talk with you about anything which may have affected . . . .'s progress in any way. She will be in touch with you to arrange a convenient date and time, and would be happy to meet you at home, or elsewhere if you would prefer it.

All information we gather on this project is confidential. No child or family is ever identified in any report, and no information would ever be passed on unless, or course, you wished.

If you have any questions please feel free to contact me. I would like to take this opportunity to thank you for your support so far in this research effort. We are very mindful of our dependence on you, and are grateful for your cooperation without which the work would be impossible.

Kindest regards.

Yours sincerely,

Phillip Bairstow,
Research Director.

Letter sent to Manchester families

7th January 1991.

Dear . . . .,

As you know, the project in which you and your child became involved during 1989 is studying the progress of selected children in the Greater Manchester area and children in the Birmingham Institute for Conductive Education. As part of this study, we need to know about anything which has been happening outside the schools which may have a bearing on the children's development. It is fairly common, for example, for children in all types of education to have help out of school. On the other hand, prolonged illness or surgery can hold a child back. It is important for us to know about these things if we are to understand how a child is progressing.

To help with this part of the study. Jeanne Downton has recently joined the research team. She has a lot of experience of working with children and families, and would like to talk with the parents of the children, starting in January 1991.

Jeanne would, therefore, like some time to talk with you about anything which may have affected . . . .'s progress in any way. She will be in touch with you shortly to arrange a convenient date and time, and would be happy to meet you at home, or at school if you would prefer it.

All information we gather on this project is confidential. No child or family is ever identified in any report, and no information would ever be passed on unless, of course, you wished.

If you have any questions please feel free to contact me. I would like to take this opportunity to thank you for your support so far in this research effort. We are very mindful of our dependence on you, and are grateful for your continuing cooperation without which the work would be impossible.

Kindest regards.

Yours sincerely,

Phillip Bairstow,
Research Director.

Appendix 6.11

Education Programme Interview: Data Sheet.

Child: Date:

Respondent:
_____

Notes:

Child:
_____

Mental Functioning

Categories of Function	Focus of the Programme			
	0	1	2	3

1. Visual short-term memory
2. Visual matching, discrimination
3. Concept formation
4. General knowledge
5. Premaths, maths
6. Time concept
7. Colour naming
8. Pre-reading, reading
9.
10.
11.
12.
_____

Child:
_____

Communication

Categories of Function	Focus of the Programme			
	0	1	2	3

1. Non-verbal comprehension
2. Non-verbal communication
3. Verbal comprehension
4. Muscle control
5. Articulation of consonants
6. Verbal expression
7.
8.
9.
10.
11.
12.
_____

Child:

Fine-Motor Functioning

Categories of Function	Focus of the Programme			
	0	1	2	3
1. Grasping, placing, releasing objects				
2. Differentiated control of fingers				
3. Two-Hand coordination				
4. Use of pencil and paper				
5. Writing				
6. Throwing and catching				
7.				
8.				
9.				
10.				
11.				
12.				

Child:

Gross-Motor Functioning

Categories of Function	Focus of the Programme			
	0	1	2	3
1. Control of static postures				
2. Position changing				
3. Crawling, creeping				
4. Walking without aids				
5. Stairs, climbing				
6. Jumping, hopping, skipping				
7. Bicycle, tricycle				
8. Skates				
9. Sports				
10.				
11.				
12.				

261

Child:

Personal Behaviour

Categories of Function	Focus of the Programme			
	0	1	2	3
1. Sense of identity				
2. Solitary activities				
3. Manners				
4. Secrets				
5. Make believe				
6. Attention span, self control				
7. Behaviour problems				
8.				
9.				
10.				
11.				
12.				

Child:

Interpersonal Behaviour

Categories of Function	Focus of the Programme			
	0	1	2	3
1. Imitation				
2. Interest in others				
3. Responsiveness to others				
4. Pleasing others				
5. Games				
6. Friendship				
7. Attending groups or clubs				
8.				
9.				
10.				
11.				
12.				

Child:

Self-Help Behaviour

Categories of Function	Focus of the Programme			
	0	1	2	3
1. Drinking				
2. Eating				
3. Dressing, undressing				
4. Toileting				
5. Washing, drying				
6. Grooming				
7. Health				
8. Preparing food				
9. Responsibility and chores				
10. Getting about				
11.				
12.				

PART II

7

7.1 INTRODUCTION

Objective 4 (Section 1.4) required a definition of the range of applicability of conductive education in Britain. This objective could be linked to Objective 3 (Section 6) in the sense that it would be worthwhile investigating the issue of 'applicability' only if conductive education were shown to be superior in effectiveness, at least in some ways, compared to United Kingdom special education. On the other hand, the Pető and Birmingham Institutes are scarcely unique among providers of education in employing a programme which has not been evaluated, and they would not be unique if they were to continue to provide conductive education regardless of the outcome of an evaluation.

The approach taken in this section, therefore, is to consider the applicability of conductive education regardless of conclusions relating to comparative effectiveness. The focus is on children with cerebral palsy because a consideration of other categories of children (Section 1.1) is outside the scope of the project. Although it was initially intended that children with disorders other than cerebral palsy (eg., spina bifida) would be admitted to the Birmingham Institute, this did not in fact happen. The following topics will be covered: reasons for rejecting children for conductive education; the rate of rejection; characteristics of children judged suitable for conductive education; comparison between rejected and accepted children. Relevant to the issue of 'applicability' is whether children in the Birmingham Institute made progress at least according to the conductors. Two further topics were, therefore, addressed: progress made by children according to conductive education assessments; agreement between conductor's records of children's progress and research assessments of their progress. An economic evaluation was outside the scope of this project.

7.2 REASONS FOR JUDGING CHILDREN UNSUITABLE FOR CONDUCTIVE EDUCATION

The process by which children were selected for the Birmingham Institute involved an incomplete screening of children within the Institute's catchment area, because not all children who would satisfy criteria in the 'Notice of Admission' (Section 6.3.1) were put forward by parents. In considering the range of possible reasons for judging children unsuitable for conductive education, it is necessary, therefore, to report data gathered during the selection of comparison children because complete samples within specified areas were screened.

Section 6.4 describes the method used to identify children with cerebral palsy who might serve as comparisons for the group enrolled at the Birmingham Institute. A total of 79 potential comparison children were put forward as satisfying a liberal interpretation of initial criteria in the Birmingham Institute's 'Notice of Admission'. Children who were not put forward, failed to satisfy one or more of these criteria, but no record was kept of the frequency with which the various criteria failed to be met. Among the children who satisfied the initial criteria, none were excluded because of lack of parental agreement but a few were unavailable for assessment for a variety of reasons like illness, absence from school, etc.

The initial criteria anticipate assessments carried out by conductors who subsequently judged 25 of the 79 potential comparison children to be unsuitable for conductive education. Another 18 children were assessed for acceptance into the Pető Institute as a control to prevent bias in the conductor's assessments and a further six of these were judged unsuitable making a total of 31.

The primary reason for rejecting 17 of the 31 children was, in the conductors' terms, a 'mental problem'. There were additional reasons for rejecting some of these children; seven were also 'microcephalic', five showed 'poor contact' with parents or conductors, four had 'visual problems', two had poorly controlled epilepsy, two showed stereotypic behaviour patterns, and two had other health problems (asthma and a cardiac problem). Some children had two or more of these additional signs. Any one of these signs when present with a 'mental problem', strengthened the case for rejecting a child for conductive education.

The term 'mental problem' is believed to be related to the 'profound mental handicap' criterion in the Birmingham Institute's 'Notice of Admission'. No independent test of cognitive functioning was carried out during the screening assessments. In the conductors' words, 'mental problem' is an exclusion criterion only when it is the primary problem from which other disabilities stem—including physical disabilities. All 66 children considered suitable for conductive education in the screening for comparisons were already in schools for the physically handicapped.

'Poor contact' is, perhaps, related to the 'autism' criterion in the 'Notice of Admission'. A judgement of 'poor contact' was made by conductors while observing a child responding to instructions and interacting with another person. If a child responded and interacted positively or negatively, the child was said to have 'good contact'. If a child generally did not respond at all to instructions and was generally indifferent, the child was said to have 'poor contact'. The conductors took into account the age of the child, and whether there was poor contact with the parents, the conductors, or both parents and conductors before arriving at an overall judgement of poor contact. Such a judgement was taken as a definite sign of a 'mental problem'.

Among the remaining 14 potential comparison children who were rejected by the conductors, two were judged unsuitable for conductive education on orthopaedic grounds. One of these children was diplegic, had an extensive history of orthopaedic surgery, and was walking with the aid of sticks. The conductors doubted whether conductive education could effect any further improvement in the child's mobility and independence. It should be noted here that orthopaedic surgery is not prohibited either as a precursor or as an adjunct to conductive education. The other child was severely athetoid and had a fixed deformity with a 5cm difference in length of her legs. Children with fixed deformities are not accepted for conductive education.

Four other children were rejected by the conductors for different reasons. One was diplegic, had recently experienced epileptic episodes, was 'hyperactive', concentrated poorly, and there was doubt as to whether the child could participate in conductive education. One child had a complicated medical picture, there was doubt about the diagnosis of cerebral palsy and there was a possibility the child had a progressive condition of some kind. Children with progressive conditions (eg., muscular dystrophy) are generally not accepted for conductive education. In another case there was also doubt about the diagnosis of cerebral palsy, with the child showing severe and generalised hypotonia. Finally, there was a case of a chronic metabolic disorder, doubt about the diagnosis of cerebral palsy, and doubt about whether the metabolic disorder could be corrected. 'Continuous ill-health' is another of the exclusion criteria for conductive education.

The remaining eight children were rejected by the conductors on the grounds that their motor problems were too mild; ie. they did not need conductive education. All eight children were currently enrolled in programmes of special education because of motor problems; four were hemiplegic, one was diplegic and three had a mild form of cerebral palsy also classed as developmental delay in the medical notes.

It is clear from the Institute's initial criteria and the results of the conductor's actual assessments that a wide variety of conditions can rule out a child with cerebral palsy for conductive education. The conditions can be grouped according to the conductor's view of their impact on conductive education.

i.   Conditions which would prevent a child from participating in conductive education, such as; low general cognitive ability, epilepsy, visual problems, deafness, any form of chronic ill-health which would prevent regular attendance.

ii. Conditions which would not prevent participation but would block improvement. For example, any form of congenital fixed physical deformity like uneven length of leg or fixed deformity of the hand. Included under this heading are fixed deformities resulting from orthopaedic surgery.

iii. Progressive conditions which would undermine possible benefits of conductive education. It is unclear whether it is believed that children with such conditions cannot benefit, or whether it is just a policy not to deal with progressive disorders. Adults with progressive conditions are accepted for conductive education; eg. Parkinson's disease.

iv. A motor condition which is so mild as not to require conductive education. All children excluded for this reason were, nevertheless, requiring special education.

It is, perhaps, obvious though nonetheless worth stating in the present context that none of the conditions just described exclude a child from special education as designed and implemented in the United Kingdom which aims to cope with the full range of children who need it. Conductive education, on the other hand, has particular requirements which demand a careful screening of potential pupils.

7.3 PREVALENCE OF CHILDREN WITH CEREBRAL PALSY JUDGED UNSUITABLE FOR CONDUCTIVE EDUCATION

In the selection of comparison children (Section 6.4), complete samples of children with cerebral palsy were effectively screened for 'suitability for conductive education' in two education authorities. According to statistics provided by the Office of Population Census and Surveys (OPCS), there is an estimated total of 75 children in the catchment areas of the authorities in the age band of this study (40–72 months on 1 January 1990) with congenital cerebral palsy. This figure is close to the local estimate of 72 children.

Of the estimated 75 children, 38 (51 per cent) satisfied Stage 1 criteria and were put forward by the local authorities. None of the parents refused their consent to the study, but some of the children could not attend the Stage 2 assessments for a variety of reasons like absence, illness, etc. Of the 32 who were available for assessment by the conductors in Stage 2, 10 (31 per cent) were considered unsuitable. Therefore, if all 38 had been assessed, it can be calculated that 12 (31 per cent of 38) would have been considered unsuitable. If these 12 children are added to the 37 who did not pass Stage 1 and the total expressed as a proportion of the estimated total number of children with cerebral palsy (75), it can be calculated that 65 per cent of children with congenital cerebral palsy aged 40–72 months are unsuitable for conductive education.

It is unlikely, for two reasons, that local authorities held back children who should have been assessed: first, authorities were actively encouraged to put forward all children who could possibly satisfy the criteria, leaving it to the conductors to apply the criteria and decide on suitability; and second, there is evidence that the authorities did apply a liberal interpretation of the criteria because children were rejected by the conductors for reasons covering the full range of known exclusion criteria.

The question arises as to whether the above estimates are in line with statistics in Hungary and whether the conductors employed criteria used at the Pető Institute. Although the research team does not have any Hungarian statistics, the blind assessment procedure employed in the present study (Section 6.4.2) was designed to ensure that criteria employed for accepting children at the Pető Institute were also employed in the present selection of children. However, the Pető Institute permits doubtful cases to be enrolled for a trial period to confirm suitability. Such cases could have been rejected in Stage 2 because the conductors knew there could not be a trial period. The Pető Institute estimates that no more than 10 per cent of all children with cerebral palsy enrolled are rejected after a trial period so it is doubtful whether an excessively conservative application of their criteria in Stage 2 could have led the conductors wrongly to exclude more than one or two children. On the other hand, some accepted comparison children's suitability is now in doubt because of their low mental ability. In all probability, the number of false negative cases equals the number of false positive cases.

The Pető Institute also accepts some very mild cases for part-time or very short-term conductive education. Such cases on this occasion may have been rejected because the conductors were effectively assessing children for full-time provision in accordance with that received by children in Birmingham. However, one of the comparison children accepted is only very mildly affected, according to all assessments, and it is difficult to envisage an even milder case needing any form of conductive education.

In summary, while the above estimate of 65 per cent non-suitability can only be taken as provisional until another independent estimate is made, there are reasons to be confident that the margin of error is small. If unsuitable children with cerebral palsy are pooled with the multitude of other excluded conditions seen in schools providing special education, it can be appreciated that conductive education could only ever be a provision for a minority of all children who need special education.

7.4 CHARACTERISTICS OF CHILDREN WITH CEREBRAL PALSY JUDGED SUITABLE FOR CONDUCTIVE EDUCATION

There is a large body of data on children enrolled in the Birmingham Institute for Conductive Education (Section 6). The group is not, however, representative of children who are suitable for conductive education for two reasons. First, all children within the Institute's catchment area who would satisfy criteria in the 'Notice of Admission' were not screened for suitability. Second, all children who were found suitable could not be accepted at the Institute and the final selection was carried out on a non-random basis.

In considering the characteristics of children who are suitable for conductive education, it is necessary to turn to data gathered during the selection of comparison children because complete samples within specified areas were screened. The body of data is, however, restricted because only a limited number of assessments were possible when large numbers of children were screened each day.

As outlined in Section 7.3 only a minority of children with cerebral palsy (35 per cent) are suitable for conductive education. The total of 54 potential comparison children passing Stage 1 and Stage 2 were judged by the conductors to be practically free of a broad range of problems and disorders that can occur with cerebral palsy including; low general cognitive ability, microcephaly, stereotypic behaviour patterns, poor contact, autistic features, epilepsy, visual problems, deafness, chronic ill health, fixed physical deformities and progressive conditions. The following additional data are available on all the children screened, including these 54 children (Table 7.1); the conductor's diagnosis and severity rating, parent report on the Self-Help, Social and Communication scales of Developmental Profile II, parent estimate of independence in 18 activities of a Gross-Motor Assessment and a direct test of preferred-hand and nonpreferred-hand function.

The most frequent diagnostic category is quadriplegia (Table 7.1) with other categories occurring in the following order of decreasing frequency; diplegia, athetosis, hemiplegia and ataxia. It would be difficult to evaluate whether the frequency of categories in this particular sample diverges from the frequency of categories in the general cerebral palsy population because of the lack of standardisation in criteria used for making diagnoses.

Children suitable for conductive education were judged by the conductors (Section 6.3.2) to be 'mild' or 'moderate' with approximately equal frequency, while there were relatively few children in the 'severe' category (Table 7.1). The fact that only 15 per cent of children passing all criteria for conductive education were judged 'severe' while 50 per cent of children enrolled in the Birmingham Institute were in the 'severe' category, shows the extent of the bias in the Birmingham sample. Part of the bias could be due to the fact that the Birmingham children were put forward by parents who were actively seeking conductive education and there is, perhaps, a tendency for parents of 'severe' children to seek alternative forms of education or therapy. This interpretation is supported by the fact that of the 'control' children accepted for the Pető Institute, that is, children put forward by parents who were actively seeking conductive education, 42 per cent were in the 'severe' category while only 8 per cent were 'mild'.

Even though conductive education is highly selective in the choice of children, other data show there is a wide range of functional abilities among those children who pass the screening procedure (Table 7.1). Perhaps 10 per cent of these children would be found unsuitable after a trial period in conductive education but that would still leave a wide range of functional abilities. Putting that issue aside, the purpose here is to report what is known about the range of abilities among the 54 children who passed the initial screening.

It can be seen in Table 7.1 that the mean developmental age of the children according to parent report on Developmental Profile II was lower than the childrens' chronological age on the Self-Help, Social and Communication scales. In addition, the children were far more variable on those scales (see standard deviations) than would be expected from the variation in chronological age.

On the Self-Help scale, one 67 month old child received a developmental age of 6 months (−61 months age-differential) indicating that the child was attempting to reach and grasp objects and would hold onto a bottle while drinking but was not able to carry out, or help with, the wide range of feeding, dressing, washing, toileting and household chore activities expected at that age. At the other extreme, a 68 month old child received a developmental age of 102 months (+34 months age-differential) with the parents claiming that the child carried out feeding, grooming and house-hold chores activities far in advance of age.

On the Social scale, a 68 month old child received a developmental age of 22 months (−46 months age-differential) because the child responded to instructions, could be engaged in solitary play, and demonstrated some attributes important for establishing interpersonal relationships but was unable to interact with adults and children, and did not show an awareness of other's feelings and possessions as would be expected at 68 months. There was, on the other hand, a 45 month old who had a developmental age of 84 months (+39 months age-differential), demonstrating superior social skills in interacting with others.

On the Communication scale, a 67 month old child received a develop-mental age of 18 months (−49 months age-differential) because the child responded to sounds and gestures for communicating but was incapable of the range of verbal communication skills expected of a 68 month old. On the other hand a 45 month old child received a developmental age of 86 months (+41 months age-differential) because it was the parent's view that the child had superior verbal skills.

There are no age-norms for the gross-motor or fine-motor assessments but it is possible, nonetheless, to indicate the range of individual abilities. Children with the severest gross-motor difficulties were incapable of independently maintaining sitting, kneeling or standing postures, incapable of independently moving between a range of postures and were incapable of any form of independent locomotion At the other extreme there were children who were fully independent on all the gross-motor items including walking (Section 6.2.7, item xvi) and the most difficult mobility task requiring standing from a high-kneeling posture (Section 6.2.7, item xiv). Children with the severest fine-motor difficulties were incapable of transferring a single ball between two trays while the most skilful child took an average of 1.6 sec to transfer each of 10 balls between two trays with the preferred-hand and an average of 1.8 sec with the non-preferred-hand.

7.5 COMPARISON BETWEEN CHILDREN JUDGED SUITABLE AND CHILDREN JUDGED UNSUITABLE FOR CONDUCTIVE EDUCATION

The 31 children judged unsuitable for conductive education during the selection of a comparison group do not form a homogenous group because there was a wide range of reasons given for rejection. It is, however, possible to identify subgroups among the 31 rejected children and to compare them to subgroups of the 66 accepted children.

As outlined in Section 7.4, the following data were among those gathered on all 97 children screened by conductors during the selection of a comparison group; conductor's severity rating, parent report on the Social and Communication scales of Developmental Profile II and parent estimate of independence in 18 activities of a Gross-Motor Assessment.

Of the 66 children accepted for conductive education, 13 were rated 'severe' by the conductors. The 17 children rejected because of a 'mental problem' would be expected to have poorly developed social and communication abilities and, perhaps, poorer abilities than the 13 children accepted but rated 'severe'. The mean chronological ages and age-differentials on the Social and Communication Scales of Developmental Profile II are given in Table 7.2. The two subgroups do not differ with respect to chronological age, but the 17 rejected children have significantly greater negative age-differentials on the Social and Communication Scale than the 13 accepted 'severe' children. The distributions do, however, overlap. There were children rejected by the conductors but not functioning as poorly according to the parents as some of the accepted children, and children accepted by the conductors but functioning just as poorly according to the parents as some of the rejected children.

Of the 66 children accepted for conductive education, 23 were rated 'mild' by the conductors. The eight children rejected because their motor problem was too mild should be more independent in 18 activities of a Gross-Motor Assessment than the 23 accepted but rated 'mild'. The mean chronological ages and the mean independence scores according to parent report on the 18 item check-list are given in Table 7.3. The two groups do not differ in chronological age, but the eight rejected children are significantly more independent than the 23 accepted 'mild' children. There were, however, several children, accepted by the conductors who were as independent according to the parents as the rejected children.

The above results show that parent report of accepted and rejected children's abilities, broadly corroborate the conductor's decision to accept or reject children, as well as the reasons given for rejection.

7.6 PROGRESS MADE BY CHILDREN ACCORDING TO THE CONDUCTOR'S ASSESSMENTS

During the period of the present study, conductors established 27 scales of development covering seven domains (Section 5.2); ie. Social Behaviour, Upper-Limb Function, Self-Care, Position Changing, Walking, Speech and Communication, Cognition. Each scale represents the conductor's view of how a child should progress in a conductive education setting.

The scales can be characterised as follows:

i.   They are metathetic scales because each step on a scale describes a behaviour which is qualitatively different from other steps.

ii. They are concerned with 'function' rather than 'ability'; ie. whether a child *does* exhibit a behaviour rather than whether a child may have an ability which is not actually used.

iii. The scales are generally not concerned with age-appropriate behaviour; ie. the age of the child is not taken into account when placing the child on a scale, and improvement in absolute terms will result in progression along the scale. There are exceptions however, and the following scales make reference to 'age-appropriate' behaviour; 'communication', 'general knowledge', 'attention', 'motivation'. On these scales, a child may improve in absolute terms but not progress along the scale unless there is improvement in relation to age.

iv. Many of the scales are concerned with the progressive acquisition of independence from physical and personal assistance in carrying out activities. The following scales are not primarily concerned with the acquisition of independence; the four Social Behaviour scales, one of the Upper Limb Function scales, the two Speech and Communication scales and the four Cognition scales. Progress on these scales may, however, promote independent functioning in other domains.

v. An attempt has been made to make the steps on the scales equidistant, and to line-up the scales within a domain so that, for example, point 8 on one scale indicates the same level of progress as point 8 on other scales. Whether this has been achieved cannot be confirmed, but the assumption will be made that the scales are interval scales of measurement.

vi. The conductors place children on the scales after a period of direct observation at the Institute in a conductive education setting. The scales are not, primarily, concerned with whether the behaviours generalise to other situations, or whether the behaviours are built into more complex behaviours. There is an exception however; 'relationship with children in play or family situation' is concerned with social behaviour in the family situation.

In order to get the conductors' view of the children's progress it was intended that the senior Hungarian conductor at the Birmingham Institute should place each child in the three intakes on their scales at the following times to coincide with research assessments (Section 6.3.5).

Time 1 Intakes 1 and 2   End 1988
          Intake 3   End 1989

Time 2 Intakes 1 and 2   End 1989
          Intake 3   End 1990

Time 3 Intakes 1 and 2   End 1990
          Intake 3   End 1991

The data set is, however, incomplete. A number of children left the Institute during the period of the study and could not be placed on the scales, and there are no Time 3 data for Intake 3 because the senior conductor doing the assessments returned to Hungary. Longitudinal Time 1, Time 2, and Time 3 data are, therefore, available on only 10 children. In addition, data in the Speech and Communication domain and the Cognition domain are incomplete because the Institute's records are not sufficiently explicit and comprehensive to enable a rating of the children. Finally, there are no Time 3 data on the 'relationships with children in play or family situation' scale because the senior conductor did not have the opportunity to visit the families to obtain the necessary information.

Table 7.4 lists the 27 conductive education scales and shows the average progress of the 10 children in the Birmingham group for which Time 1, Time 2 and Time 3 data are available. Missing data in the table indicate incomplete records even for these 10 children. Section 5.2 can be consulted for an explanation of what the data means in terms of function.

Overall, the children showed a modest and steady improvement on eight of the scales. On the remaining 13 scales for which Time 1, Time 2 and Time 3 data are available, the children showed either no overall improvement, a plateau at Time 3 or a deterioration at Time 3. Greatest overall improvement was shown on the 'toileting' scale while least improvement was shown on the 'walking without aids' scale.

Data in Table 7.4 conceal differences between children in their progress on the scales. Considering change over the period Time 1 to Time 3, there were individuals who showed greater progress on each of the scales than the group average. On the other hand, for 15 scales there were children showing no improvement and on two scales there were children who deteriorated. On only five scales did all 10 children perform better at Time 3 than Time 1; ie., 'feeding', 'toileting', 'standing up from a stool and sitting down to a stool', 'standing up from the floor and sitting down to the floor', 'walking with aids'.

7.7 AGREEMENT BETWEEN CONDUCTOR'S RECORDS OF CHILDREN'S PROGRESS AND RESEARCH ASSESSMENTS OF THEIR PROGRESS

7.7.1 Introduction

It is first necessary to establish whether there is commonality between conductive education scales and any of the research scales in terms of their characteristics and content. Where commonality exists, agreement between conductor's assessments and research assessments can be investigated.

Wherever possible, research scales involving direct testing and observation will be used as parallels for the conductive education scales because the latter also involve direct observation of children. Where there is no research scale involving direct testing, indirect assessments involving interviews with conductors and other staff of the Birmingham Institute will be chosen because the data will be relevant to the behaviour of the children in the Institute.

The research scales and the conductive education scales are generally not closely parallel. The research scales include most of the types of items which are to be found in the conductive education scales, but also cover a far wider range of behaviours. There are, however, a few items in the conductive education scales which cannot be found in the research scales. It is necessary, at times, to regroup some of the research scales for the present purpose to make the research data closer in nature to the conductive education data. It is necessary also to pool data across conductive education scales because there is usually no research parallel to individual conductive education scale. This pooling is possible because the scales were constructed so that consecutive points on a scale are equidistant and scales within a domain 'line-up' so that, for example, point 5 on one scale is developmentally equivalent to point 5 on other scales (Section 7.6).

The following analyses will concern only those children at the Institute who were assessed by the senior Hungarian conductor; ie. 17 children at Time 1 and Time 2 and 10 children at Time 3 (Section 7.6).

7.7.2   Social Behaviour

The four conductive education scales in this domain are, broadly speaking, concerned with interpersonal relationships; ie., the way the child behaves in a group, relates to adults and children, and initiates social contact (Section 5.2). There is no parallel among the research assessments to any one of these scales but there is for the four scales combined, hence data were pooled across the scales at Time 1 and Time 2. There is no summation of data for Time 3 because one of the social scales was not completed by the senior Hungarian conductor. The difference between the sum of Time 2 and Time 1 scores was calculated for each child, and this difference is an overall measure of progress made along the social scales.

The research team carried out no direct assessment of social behaviour of the children, but conductors and other Institute staff were interviewed about their view of the childrens' behaviour at the Institute. The Interpersonal Relationships scale of the Vineland Adaptive Behaviour Scales used for the interview with conductors is similar to the conductive education scales in as much as it is a metathetic scale, concerned with function rather than ability and the items are not concerned with 'age-related' behaviour. In addition, an interval scale is implied because each item 'passed' contributes equally to a raw score sum. Finally, most of the items are concerned with interpersonal relationships, but there are some additional items dealing with personal behaviour and communication. Childrens' behaviour within the Institute was being assessed because that is the environment in which the conductor had most experience observing the children. The raw score at Time 1 and Time 2 for each child and the difference between Time 2 and Time 1 scores are used in the present analyses.

There are significant correlations between the conductor's assessment of the social behaviour of the children and the research assessment of the children at Time 1 and Time 2, but there is poor agreement between the Time 2–Time 1 measure of progress (Table 7.5).

7.7.3   Upper Limb Function

The six conductive education scales in this domain, three each for the right and left limb, are concerned with finger movement, manipulation, grasping and reaching (Section 5.2). There is no parallel among research assessments to any one of these scales but there is for a combination of the scales, hence data were pooled across the scales for each child at Time 1, Time 2 and Time 3. The difference between Time 2 and Time 1 and between Time 3 and Time 1 scores was calculated. These differences are overall measures of progress made along the upper limb function scales.

The research team carried out a direct assessment of upper limb function. There were two tasks which encompass functions assessed by the conductive education scales. The 'peg-board' task (Section 6.2.6.2) requires the transfer of pegs from one line of holes in a board to another line of holes, using the right and left hand. The 'ball-transfer' task (Section 6.2.6.3) requires the transfer of balls of varying size and weight from one tray to another tray, using the right and left hand. Differentiated movements of the fingers is required in picking up the pegs and balls which vary in size, shape and weight. Grasping objects of various size, shape and weight is required in transporting the objects to the target location. Both tasks require reaching in a variety of directions in order to pick up objects in various locations and then to transport them to various target locations. Manipulation is required in the pegboard task to orientate the peg and to place it in the target hole. In each task, the number of objects transferred is divided by the total time taken to perform the task to arrive at the measure of 'rate of transfer'. The higher the 'rate of transfer' the more skilful the overall performance. A combination of the two right-limb and two left-limb scales is similar to the conductive education scales in as much as it is concerned with function rather than ability and are not concerned with 'age-related' behaviour. In addition, the children are directly assessed and the abilities measured are similar to those observed in the conductive education scales. The research scales differ from the conductive education scales in that the former are prosthetic scales while the latter are metathetic scales. The mean 'rate of transfer' of objects at Time 1, Time 2 and Time 3, and the difference between Time 2 and Time 1 and between Time 3 and Time 1 was calculated.

There are significant correlations between the conductor's assessment of the upper limb function of the children and the research assessment of the children at Time 1, Time 2 and Time 3 but poor agreement between the Time 2–Time 1 and Time 3–Time 1 measures of progress (Table 7.5).

7.7.4   Self-Care

The five conductive education scales in this domain are concerned with putting on and taking off clothes and footwear, tying and untying shoelaces, doing up and undoing buttons, use of cutlery in feeding as well as chewing and swallowing, toileting including indicating the need and use of potty, toilet and toilet paper (Section 5.2). There is no parallel among research assessments to any one of these scales but there is for five scales combined, hence data are pooled across the scales for each child at Time 1, Time 2 and Time 3. The difference between Time 2 and Time 1 and between Time 3 and Time 1 scores was calculated. These differences are overall measures of progress made along the self-care scales.

The research team carried out no direct assessment of self-care behaviour of the children, but conductors were interviewed about their view of the childrens' behaviour using the Activities of Daily Living scale (Section 6.2.9.4) of the Vineland Adaptive Behaviour Scales. This scale is similar to the conductive education scales in as much as it is a metathetic scale, concerned with function rather than ability and the items are not concerned with 'age-related' behaviour. In addition, an interval scale is implied because each item contributes equally to a raw score, and items are concerned with putting on and taking off clothes, tying and untying shoe laces, use of fasteners and zippers, use of cutlery in feeding as well as chewing, toileting including indicating the need and use of potty and toilet. The Vineland scale differs from the conductive education scales mainly in that the former covers a wider range of behaviours such as bathing, drying the body, toothwash, nose care, grooming and health care. The raw score for Time 1, Time 2 and Time 3 for each child and the difference between Time 2 and Time 1 and between Time 3 and Time 1 are used in the present analyses.

There are significant correlations between the conductor's assessment of the self-care of the children and the research assessment of the children at Time 1, Time 2 and Time 3 but there is poor agreement between the Time 2–Time 1 and Time 3–Time 1 measures of progress (Table 7.5).

7.7.5   Position Changing and Walking

The four conductive education scales in the domain of Position Changing are concerned with posture and mobility, but not with locomotion. They cover the following activities; standing up from a stool, sitting down to a stool, standing up from the floor, sitting down to the floor, standing, sitting up from supine, lying down to supine, sitting on the plinth, and sideways rolling on the floor. The two conductive education scales in the domain of Walking are concerned with standing barefoot, walking barefoot and without aids on a variety of surfaces, and walking with aids on a variety of surfaces. There is no annual research assessment like any of these individual scales but there is one for six scales combined, hence data are pooled across the scales for each child at Time 1, Time 2 and Time 3. The difference between Time 2 and Time 1 and between Time 3 and Time 1 was calculated.

While there was no annual direct research assessment of gross motor function there was an annual indirect assessment. Conductors and other staff at the Birmingham Institute were interviewed about their view of the childrens' functioning using the Gross-Motor Scale of the Vineland Adaptive Behaviour Scales. This scale is similar to the combination of conductive education scales in as much as it is a metathetic scale concerned with function rather than ability and the items are not concerned with 'age-related' behaviour. An interval scale is implied because each item contributes equally to a raw score. While there are items concerned with sitting, sitting up from supine, standing up and walking, the Vineland scale differs in content and is broader than the conductive education scales; the former has items concerned with crawling, running, jumping, use of stairs, climbing, hopping, throwing, catching, use of tricycle and bicycle, while the latter have additional items concerned with mobility and locomotion. Despite these differences there is perhaps sufficient commonality between the Vineland scale and the combination of the six conductive education scales for a parallel to be drawn. The raw score for Time 1, Time 2 and Time 3 for each child and the difference between Time 2 and Time 1 and between Time 3 and Time 1 are used in the present analyses.

There are significant correlations between the conductors assessments of position-changing and walking and the research assessment at Time 1, Time 2 and Time 3 but there is poor agreement between the Time 2–Time 1 and Time 3–Time 1 measures of progress (Table 7.5).

There was a direct research assessment of gross-motor function at Time 1 and Time 3. One part of the assessment had items similar in nature to activities covered by the four Position Changing scales; standing up from the floor (prone to four point kneeling (Section 6.2.7, ix), to high kneeling (Section 6.2.7, xii), to standing (Section 6.2.7., xiv)) lying down to supine (Section 6.2.7, iv), and sideways rolling on the floor (Section 6.2.7., vi & vii). For each item the speed at which the activity is carried out is calculated. The research scales differ from the conductive education scale in that the former are prosthetic scales while the latter are metathetic scales.

There are significant correlations between the conductor's assessment of position changing and the research assessment at Time 1 and Time 3 but poor agreement between Time 3–Time 1 measure of progress (Table 7.5).

Part of the direct research assessment of gross-motor function at Time 1 and Time 3 required walking barefoot with assistance from a helper if necessary (Section 6.2.7, xvi). The speed at which a set distance is covered was calculated. This item has similarities to the 'Walking: without aids and barefoot' conductive education scale, except that the research scale is a prosthetic scale while the conductive education scale is a metathetic scale.

There are significant correlations between the conductor's assessment of walking and the research assessment at Time 1 and Time 3 but poor agreement between Time 3–Time 1 measure of progress (Table 7.5).

7.7.6 Speech and Communication

The Hungarian conductor was able to rate the children at Time 1, Time 2 and Time 3 only on the speech scale.

The research team carried out a direct assessment of speech and communication. Assessment of the production of sounds in isolation (10 items in the Dysarthria Assessment), the production of syllable strings (5 items in the Dysarthria Assessment), the articulation of consonants in isolated words (Edinburgh Articulation Test), and language structure (part of the Reynell Expressive Language Scale), are related to functions assessed by the conductive education Speech scale. In addition, the research scales are similar to the conductive education scale in as much as they are metathetic scales concerned with function, the items are not concerned with 'age-appropriate' behaviour, and interval scales are implied because each item contributes equally to a raw score sum. The sum of raw scores on the above tests for each child at Time 1, Time 2 and Time 3 and the difference between Time 2 and Time 1 and between Time 3 and Time 1 are used in the present analyses.

There are significant correlations between the conductor's assessment of speech and the research assessments at Time 1, Time 2 and Time 3 but poor agreement between Time 2—Time 1 and Time 3—Time 1 measures of progress (Table 7.5).

The research scales which are closest in content to the conductive education Communication scale are six Pre-verbal Communication Scales and part of the Reynell Expressive Language Scale (Language Content). As already pointed out, the conductive education scale takes into account the age of the child and a child cannot progress along the scale unless progress exceeds the average for the age group (Section 7.6). The Pre-verbal Communication Scales, however, do not take into account the age of the child, hence it is improper to draw any parallels between the assessments. While items in the Reynell Expressive Language Scale also do not take into account the age of the child, the total raw score for the three sections of the scale can be converted to a standard score by reference to tables. This standard score comes close, in nature, to the raw score obtained on the conductive education scale but the Reynell Expressive Language age equivalent is relevant not only to the content of Language but also to language structure and verbal vocabulary. In addition, the Reynell scale is not concerned with non-verbal communication. In short there is no research scale which comes close in content and nature to the conductive education scale.

7.7.7 Cognition

The conductor was unable to rate the children on any of the four scales in this domain at Time 1 and Time 2. Even if this had been possible, there are few parallels among the research assessments to any of the conductive education scales.

The General Knowledge scale is concerned with the child's knowledge of personal and impersonal circumstances. Most of the items imply an assessment of age appropriate behaviour; hence, a child cannot progress along the scale unless progress exceeds the average for the group.

The Pictorial Test of Intelligence is a direct test of cognition carried out by the research staff. Some items of the Information and Comprehension scale of this test are similar in content to the General Knowledge scale, but the former scale, as a whole, is broader in scope. Only an age equivalent can be obtained from the Information and comprehension scale; hence, a child can make progress on the scale even if progress does not exceed the average for the age group. The conductive education and research scale are, therefore, not similar.

The Attention conductive education scale is concerned with the attention of the child in a variety of circumstances. Some items at the top of the scale imply an assessment of age appropriate behaviour; hence a child cannot be placed at the top of the scale unless attention is better than average.

While the research team also carries out an assessment of attention by interviewing conductors about the behaviour of the children, the research scale is not concerned with age appropriate behaviour. The conductive education and research scales are, therefore, not similar.

The Learning Ability conductive education scale is concerned with ability to learn and ability to use what has been newly acquired in the context of what has been previously learned. The items do not require reference to the age of a child; hence, a child can progress along the scale if there is an absolute improvement in 'learning ability' but no improvement in relation to other children of the same age.

It is commonly believed that general tests of cognition assess mental abilities relevant to 'learning ability'. The Pictorial Test of Intelligence employed by the research team yields a general index of mental ability in the form of 'mental age'. A child can progress on the mental scale even if there is no improvement in relation to other children of the same age.

There is, perhaps, sufficient commonality in the nature and characteristics of the conductive education scale and the Mental Age research scale for a parallel to be drawn, but the group leader was unable to provide ratings for the children.

The Motivation conductive education scale is concerned with the self-motivation of the child. There is no research scale of similar nature and characteristics.

7.7.8 Summary

There was sufficient commonality between conductor's scales of development and research scales in most domains (social behaviour, upper limb function, self-care, position changing and walking, speech) to permit an investigation of agreement between conductor assessments and research assessments of the children. There was good agreement between the rank ordering of children at Time 1, Time 2 and Time 3, but poor agreement between the two assessments in how the children were rank ordered on progress.

Some children showed a marked progression along the conductive education scales but little change on the research scales. On the other hand, children sometimes regressed on the research scales but this rarely happened on the conductive education scales. The intervals on the conductor's scales are, perhaps, smaller than on the research scales, hence, large advances on the former do not necessarily show in advances on the latter.

The nature of the conductive education scales detailed in Section 5.2 and the above analyses suggest that when conductors refer to large advances in the abilities of individual children, they are observing progress which may not be apparent without close observation and the assistance of measuring instruments with very small intervals between steps on the scales.

7.8 Conclusions

i.   A wide range of clinical conditions and functional characteristics can lead to a child being judged by the conductors as unsuitable for conductive education.

ii. The Pető Institute's screening procedure, employing non-standardized criteria, rejects for conductive education an estimated 65 per cent of children with congential cerebral palsy. Pooling these children with the wide range of other childhood conditions which are not accepted, it seems that conductive education is, at best, suitable for only a minority of children with motor disorders.

iii. While conductive education has particular requirements in terms of the type of child that can be accepted into the programme, there is a wide range of abilities among the children who are acceptable.

iv.   Children within some categories of rejection have been found to differ significantly from children accepted for conductive education on independent tests of function. It is theoretically possible, therefore, to establish objective criteria for acceptance based on test results rather than the currently prevailing system of judgement.

v.   Relevant to the issue of 'applicability' is the finding that children at the Birmingham Institute, as a group, made only modest progress over a two year period on the conductor's own scales of development and there were signs of plateauing below the ceiling on a range of scales. On the other hand, a small number of children showed marked improvement on some of the scales, while there were other children who showed no improvement on some scales.

vi.   There is poor agreement between progress made by children on the conductor's scales of development and progress on the research scales. Generally, progress of children observed by conductors would be difficult to see without close observation and the assistance of very sensitive measuring instruments.

vii.   Data gathered from the conductor's own assessments must be regarded as disappointing in the light of claims made on behalf of conductive education by its proponents, and do not appear to justify the widespread introduction of the system into the Untied Kingdom.

Table 7.1 Data on 54 children who passed all screening assessments and were judged suitable for conductive education by staff from the Pető Institute.

Variable		54 children judged suitable for conductive education
Conductor's Diagnosis (Quad. Di. Athet. At. Hemi.)		25:12:8:3:6
Conductor's Severity Rating (Sev. Mod. Mild)		8:24:22
Chronological Age†	Mean	51.7
	SD	9.9
Developmental Profile II†		
Self-help scale	Mean	36.4
	SD	18.9
Social scale	Mean	44.8
	SD	18.5
Communication scale	Mean	45.3
	SD	22.5
Gross-Motor Independence	Mean	41.2
	SD	9.8
Fine-Motor Function*		
Preferred-hand	Mean	0.27
	SD	0.16
Nonpreferred-hand	Mean	0.19
	SD	0.16

† Months
* balls/sec

Table 7.2 Data on children judged suitable and unsuitable for conductive education. All ages are in months.

Developmental Profile II	Suitable Severe (N=13)		Unsuitable 'Mental Problem' (N=17)		Comparison	
	M	SD	M	SD	t	p
Chronological Age	48.7	10.6	56.5	18.2	1.37	ns
Social Age Differential	−19.3	8.3	−33.7	18.5	2.61	p<.02
Communication Age Differential	−17.7	22.0	−38.4	21.5	2.59	p<.02

Table 7.3 Data on children judged suitable and unsuitable for conductive education.

	Suitable Mild (N=23)		Unsuitable 'Too Mild' (N=8)		Comparison	
	M	SD	M	SD	t	p
Chronological Age	52.1	8.8	47.4	7.6	1.35	ns
Gross-Motor Independence Score	49.0	3.2	53.0	1.1	3.43	p<.01

Table 7.4 **Average Score on conductive education scales of 10 children in the Birmingham Institute for which Time 1, Time 2 and Time 3 data are available.**

Domain	Scale	Time		
		1	**2**	**3**
Social behaviour	Formal group role	5	6	6
	Relationships with adults	6	7	7
	Relationships with children	5	7	—
	Initiating individual contact	6	7	7
Right upper-limb function	Movement of fingers	5	6	6
	Reaching	5	6	6
	Holding an object	6	7	6
Left upper-limb function	Movement of fingers	5	6	7
	Reaching	5	6	7
	Holding an object	6	7	7
Self-care	Dressing	3	4	5
	Shoelaces	3	4	4
	Buttons	3	4	3
	Feeding	4	5	6
	Toileting	3	5	6
Position changing	Stool	4	5	6
	Floor	3	4	5
	Plinth	3	5	5
	Rolling	5	6	6
Walking	Without aids	6	6	6
	With aids	4	5	6
Speech and communication	Speech	6	7	7
	Communication	—	—	—
Cognition	General knowledge	—	—	—
	Attention	—	—	—
	Learning ability	—	—	—
	Motivation	—	—	—

Table 7.5 Correlations† between conductor's assessment and research assessment of children in the Birmingham Institute at Time 1, Time 2 and Time 3 together with correlations for Time 2–Time 1 and Time 3–Time 1 measure of progress.

Domain		Time 1	Time 2	3	Time 2–1	Time 3–1
Social behaviour	r_s	0.53*	0.69**	—	0.38	—
	N	17	17	—	17	—
Upper limb function	r_s	0.75**	0.72**	0.85**	−0.35	−0.03
	N	17	17	10	17	10
Self-care	r_s	0.80**	0.90**	0.64*	0.25	−0.42
	N	17	17	10	17	10
Position changing and walking (indirect assessment)	r_s	0.71**	0.91**	0.55*	−0.13	−0.08
	N	17	17	10	17	10
Position changing (direct assessment)	r_s	0.69**	—	0.66*	—	−0.04
	N	17	—	10	—	10
Walking (direct assessment)	r_s	0.48*	—	0.74*	—	0.44
	N	17	—	10	—	10
Speech	r_s	0.63**	0.79**	0.69*	0.25	0.39
	N	16	17	10	16	10

† Spearman rank correlation coefficient
* p<.05
** p<.01

References

Abbott, R., Forem, S. L. and Johann, M. (1989). Selective posterior rhizotomy for the treatment of spasticity—a review. *Child's Nervous System*, **5**, 337–346.

Akos, K. (1975). *Scientific Studies in Conductive Pedagogy*. Institute of Conductive Education of the Motor Disabled: Budapest.

Alpern, G., Boll, T. and Shearer, M. (1986). *Developmental Profile II*. Western Psychological Services: Los Angeles.

Anthony, A., Bogle, D., Ingram, T. T. S. and McIsaac, M. W. (1971). *The Edinburgh Articulation Test*. Churchill Livingstone: London.

Bairstow, P. J. (1983). Development of Motor Skills. In: R. Harre and R. Lamb (Eds). *Encyclopedic Dictionary of Psychology*. Blackwell: Oxford, 147–149.

Banich, M. T., Levine S. C., Kim, H. and Huttenlocher, P. (1990). The effects of developmental factors on IQ in hemiplegic children. *Neuropsychologica*, **28**, 35–47.

Bax, M. C. O. (1986). Aims and outcomes of therapy for the cerebral-palsied child. *Developmental Medicine and Child Neurology*, **28**, 695–696.

Bax, M. C. O. and Brown, J. K. (1985). Contractures and their therapy. *Developmental Medicine and Child Neurology*, **27**, 423–424.

Blair, E. and Stanley F. (1985). Interobserver agreement in the classification of cerebral palsy. *Developmental Medicine and Child Neurology*, **27**, 615–622.

Blake, D. D., Andrasik, F., McCarran, M. and Quinn, S. (1985). Validity of six measures for assessing social skills in cerebral-palsied patients. *Developmental Medicine and Child Neurology*, **27**, 98.

Bleck, E. E. (1975). Locomotor prognosis in cerebral palsy. *Developmental Medicine and Child Neurology*, **17**, 18–25.

Bleck, E. E. (1990). Factors effecting independence of the physically disabled. *Developmental Medicine and Child Neurology*, **32**, 189–190.

Bolanos, A. A., Bleck, E. E., Firestone, P. and Young, L. (1989). Comparison of stereognosis and two-point discrimination testing of the hands of children with cerebral palsy. *Developmental Medicine and Child Neurology*, **31**, 371–376.

Bourget, C. C., McArtor, R. E. and Roolstown, G. (1989). Physiotherapy for children with cerebral palsy. *American Journal of Diseases of Childhood*, **143**, 552–555.

Brown, J. K., Van Rensburg, F., Walsh, G., Lakie, M. and Wright, G. W. (1987). A neurological study of hand function of hemiplegic children. *Developmental Medicine and Child Neurology*, **29**, 287–304.

Classification of Occupations and Coding Index (1980). Her Majesty's Stationery Office: London.

Cooke, P. H., Cole, W. G. and Carey, R. P. L. (1989). Dislocation of the hip in cerebral palsy. *Journal of Bone and Joint Surgery*, **71**, 441–446.

Coop, R. H., Eckel, E. and Stuck, G. B. (1975). An assessment of the Pictorial Test of Intelligence for use with young cerebral palsied children. *Developmental Medicine and Child Neurology*, **17**, 287–292.

Cooper, D. (1986). "A special kind of magic": changes in family dynamics arising from parent participation in a conductive education programme for children with cerebral palsy. *Community Health Studies*, **10**, 294–306.

Corbett, J. and Loring, A. (1989). Innovations in the management of children with profound cerebral palsy and head injury. *Journal of the Royal Society of Medicine*, **82**, 634.

Cottam, P. J. and Sutton, A. (1986). *Conductive Education: A System for Overcoming Motor Disorder*. Croom Helm: London.

Cotton, E. (1965). The Institute for Movement Therapy and School for 'Conductors', Budapest, Hungary. *Developmental Medicine and Child Neurology*, **7**, 437–446.

Cotton, E. (1986). *Conductive Education and Cerebral Palsy*. The Spastics Society: London.

Craft, M. J., Lakin, J. A., Oppliger, R. A., Clancy, G. M. and Vanderlinden, D. W. (1990). Siblings as change agents for promoting the functional status of children with cerebral palsy. *Developmental Medicine and Child Neurology*, **32**, 1049–1057.

Craig, C. L. and Zimbler, S. (1990). Orthopaedic procedures. In: M. B. Glenn and J. Whyte (Eds). *The Practical Management of Spasticity in Children and Adults*. Lea and Febiger: London, 268–295.

Deluca, P. A. (1991). Gait analysis in the treatment of the ambulatory child with cerebral palsy. *Clinical Orthopaedics and Related Research*, **264**, 65–75.

Diamond, M. (1986). Rehabilitation strategies for the child with cerebral palsy. *Pediatric Annals*, **15**, 230–236.

Enderby, P. M. (1983). *Frenchay Dysarthria Assessment*. NFER–Nelson: Windsor.

Evans, P. M. and Alberman, E. (1985). Recording motor defects of children with cerebral palsy. *Developmental Medicine and Child Neurology*, **27**, 401–406.

Evans, P. M. and Alberman, E. (1990). Certified cause of death in children and young adults with cerebral palsy. *Archives of Disease in Childhood*, **55**, 325–329.

Evans, P., Elliott, M., Alberman, E. and Evans, S. (1985). Prevalence and disabilities in 4 to 8 year olds with cerebral palsy. *Archives of Disease in Childhood*, **60**, 940–945.

Farmer, S. F., Harrison, L. M., Ingram, D. A. and Stephans, J. A. (1991). Plasticity of central motor pathways in children with hemiplegic cerebral palsy. *Neurology*, **41**, 1505–1510.

Feldman, P. A. (1990). Upper extremity casting and splinting. In: M. B. Glenn and J. Whyte (Eds). *The Practical Management of Spasticity in Children and Adults*. Lea and Febiger: London, 149–166.

Fernandez, J. E., Pitetti, K. H. and Betzen, M. T. (1990). Physiological capacities of individuals with cerebral palsy. *Human Factors*, **32**, 457–466.

Fletcher (1978). *The Fletcher Time-by-Count Test of Diadochokinetic Syllable Rate*. C. C. Publications: Oregon.

French, J. L. (1964). *Pictorial Test of Intelligence*. Houghton Mifflin: Boston.

Gage, J. R. (1983). Gait analysis for decision-making in cerebral palsy. *Bulletin of the Hospital for Joint Diseases Orthopaedic Institute*, **43**, 147–163.

Gans, B. M. and Glenn, M. B. (1990). Introduction. In: M. B. Glenn and J. Whyte (Eds). *The Practical Management of Spasticity in Children and Adults*. Lea and Febiger: London, 1–7.

Giebler, K. B. (1990). Physical modalities. In: M. B. Glenn and J. Whyte (Eds). *The Practical Management of Spasticity in Chidren and Adults*. Lea and Febiger: London, 118–148.

Glenn, M. B. (1990). Nerve blocks. In: M. B. Glenn and J. Whyte (Eds). *The Practical Management of Spasticity in Children and Adults*. Lea and Febiger: London, 227–258.

Goldkamp, O. (1984). Treatment effectiveness in cerebral palsy. *Archives of Physical Medicine and Rehabilitation*, **65**, 232–234.

H. M. Inspectors (1989). *Educating Physically Disabled Pupils*. Department of Education and Science: London.

Hagberg, B., Hagberg, G. and Zetterstrom, R. (1989). Decreasing perinatal mortality—increase in cerebral palsy morbidity? *Acta Paediatrica Scandinavica*, **78**, 664–670.

Hallenborg, S. C. (1990). Positioning. In: M. B. Glenn and J. Whyte (Eds). *The Practical Management of Spasticity in Children and Adults*. Lea and Febiger: London, 97–117.

Hanzlik, J. R. (1990). Nonverbal interaction patterns of mothers and their infants with cerebral palsy. *Education and Training in Mental Retardation*, **25**, 333–343.

Hari, M. (1968). *Address Given on Conductive Education*. Castle Priory College, Wallingford, Oxford.

Hari, M. (1975). The idea of learning in conductive pedagogy. In: K. Akos (Ed). *Scientific Studies on conductive Pedagogy*. Institute of Conductive Education of the Motor Disabled: Budapest, 10–17.

Hari, M. and Akos, K. (1988). *Conductive Education*. Routledge: London.

Hari, M. and Tillemans, T. (1984). Conductive education. In: D. Scrutton (Ed). *Management of the Motor Disorders of Children with Cerebral Palsy*. Spastics International Medical Publications: London, 19–35.

Hill, L. D. (1985). Contributions of behaviour modification to cerebral palsy habilitation. *Physical Therapy*, **65**, 341–345.

Hinderer, K. A., Harris, S. R., Purdy, A. H., Chew, D. E., Staheli, L. T., McLaughlin, J. F. and Jaffe, K. M. (1988). Effects of 'tone-reducing' vs standard plaster-casts on gait improvement of children with cerebral palsy. *Developmental Medicine and Child Neurology*, **30**, 370–377.

Holm, V. A., Harthun-Smith, L. and Tada, W. L. (1983). Infant walkers and cerebral palsy. *American Journal of Diseases in Childhood*, **137**, 1189–1190.

Holt, K. S. (1981). Review: the assessment of walking in children with particular reference to cerebral palsy. *Child: Care, Health and Development*, **7**, 281–297.

Hylton, N. (1990). Dynamic casting and orthotics. In: M. B. Glenn and J. Whyte (Eds). *The Practical Management of Spasticity in Children and Adults*. Lea and Febiger: London, 167–200.

Jarvis, S. and Hey, E. (1984). Measuring disability and handicap due to cerebral palsy. In: F. Stanley and E. Alberman (Eds). *The Epidemiology of Cerebral Palsy: Clinics in Developmental Medicine, No. 87*. Blackwell: Oxford, 35–45.

Jernqvist, L. (1986). Conductive education: an education system for children with neurological disorders. *European Journal of Special Needs Education*, **1**, 3–12.

Kanda, T., Yuge, M., Yamori, Y., Suzuki, J. and Fukase, H. (1984). Early physiotherapy in the treatment of spastic diplegia. *Developmental Medicine and Child Neurology*, **26**, 438–444.

Karlsson, B., Nauman, B. and Gardestrom, L. (1960). Results of physical treatment in cerebral palsy. *Cerebral Palsy Bulletin*, **2**, 278–285.

Kiernan, C. and Reid, B. (1987). *Pre-verbal Communication Schedule*. NFER–Nelson: Windsor.

Krasner, P. R. and Siverstein, L. (1976). The preschool attainment record: a concurrent validity study with cerebral palsied children. *Educational and Psychological Measurement*, **36**, 1049–1054.

Larsson, L. E., Miller, M., Norlin, R. and Tkaczuk, H. (1986). Changes in gait patterns after operations in children with spastic cerebral palsy. *International Orthopaedics*, **10**, 155–162.

Laskas, C. A., Mullen, S. L., Nelson, D. L. and Wilson-Broyles, M. (1985). Enhancement of two motor functions of the lower extremity in a child with spastic quadriplegia. *Physical Therapy*, **65**, 11–16.

Laszlo, J. I. and Bairstow, P. J. (1985). *Perceptual-Motor Behaviour: Developmental Assessment and Therapy*. Holt, Rinehart and Winston: London.

Law, M. and Letts, L. (1989). A critical review of scales of activities of daily living. *The American Journal of Occupational Therapy*, **43**, 522–528.

Lee, D. N., Turnbull, J. and Cook, M. L. (1989). Disorder of felt position of parts of the body in hemiparetic cerebral palsied children. *International Journal of Rehabilitation Research*, **12**, 90–93.

Leonard, C. T., Moritani, T., Hirschfeld, H. and Forssberg, H. (1990). Deficits in reciprocal inhibition of children with cerebral palsy as revealed by H reflex testing. *Developmental Medicine and Child Neurology*, **32**, 974–984.

Lesny, I., Nachtmann, M., Stehlik, A., Tomankova, A., and Zajidkova, J. (1990). Disorders of memory of motor sequences in cerebral palsied children. *Brain and Development*, **12**, 339–341.

Lonton, A. P. and Russell, A. (1989). Conductive education—magic or myth? Presented at 33rd meeting of the *Society for Research into Hydrocephalus and Spina Bifida*, Cambridge.

Magill-Evans, J. E. and Restall, G. (1991). Self-esteem of persons with cerebral palsy: from adolescence to adulthood. *American Journal of Occupational Therapy*, **45**, 819–825.

Mayberry, W. and Gilligan, M. B. (1985). Ocular pursuit in mentally retarded, cerebral palsied, and learning disabled children. *American Journal of Occupational Therapy*, **39**, 589–595.

McCarty, S. M., St. James, P., Berninger, V. W. and Gans, B. M. (1986). Assessment of intellectual functioning across the life-span in severe cerebral palsy. *Developmental Medicine and Child Neurology*, **28**, 364–374.

McPherson, J. J., Schild, R., Spaulding, S. J., Barsamian, P., Transon, C. and White, S. C. (1991). Analysis of upper extremity movement in four sitting positions: a comparison of persons with and without cerebral palsy. *American Journal of Occupational Therapy*, **45**, 123–129.

Myhr, U. and von Wendt, L. (1991). Improvement of functional sitting position for children with cerebral palsy. *Developmental Medicine and Child Neurology*, **33**, 246–256.

Nash, J., Neilson, P. D. and O'Dwyer, N. J. (1989). Reducing spasticity to control muscle contracture of children with cerebral palsy. *Developmental Medicine and Child Neurology*, **31**, 471–480.

Nelson, K. B. and Ellenberg, J. H. (1982). Children who 'outgrew' cerebral palsy. *Pediatrics*, **69**, 529–536.

Norlin, R. and Odenrick, P. (1986). Development of gait in spastic children with cerebral palsy. *Journal of Pediatric Orthopaedics*, **6**, 674–680.

O'Donoghue, P. (1988). Relaxation in cerebral palsy. *Developmental Medicine and Child Neurology*, **30**, 115–117.

O'Dwyer, N. J., Neilson, P. D. and Nash, J. (1989). Mechanisms of muscle growth related to muscle contracture in cerebral palsy. *Developmental Medicine and Child Neurology*, **31**, 543–547.

Office of the Santa Cruz County Superintendent of Schools. *Behavioral Characteristics Progression*. VORT Corporation: Palo Alto.

Plamer, F. B., Shapiro, B. K., Wachtel, R. C., Allen, M. C., Hiller, J. E., Harryman, S. E., Mosher, B. S., Meinert, C. C. and Capute, A. J. (1988). The effects of physical therapy on cerebral palsy. *The New England Journal of Medicine*, **318**, 803–808.

Parette, H. P., Holder, L. F. and Sears, J. D. (1984). Correlates of therapeutic progress by infants with cerebral palsy and motor delay. *Perceptual and Motor Skills*, **58**, 159–163.

Parette, H. P. and Hourcade, J. J. (1984). How effective are physiotherapeutic programmes with young mentally retarded children who have cerebral palsy. *Journal of Mental Deficiency Research*, **28**, 167–175.

Patrick, J. (1989). Cerebral Palsy diplegia: improvements for walking. *British Medical Journal*, **299**, 1115–1116.

Peacock, W. J. and Staudt, L. A. (1991). Functional outcomes following selective posterior rhizotomy in children with cerebral palsy. *Journal of Neurosurgery*, **74**, 380–385.

Pearson, L. (1991). The conductive education movement in the UK. *NSW Journal of Special Education*, **14**, 31–39.

Phelps, W. M. (1990). Cerebral birth injuries: their orthopaedic classification and subsequent treatment. *Clinical Orthopaedics and Related Research*, **253**, 4–11.

Presland, J. (1991). Undertaking conductive education: reflections on a visit to Kiskunhalas. *NSW Journal of Special Education*, **14**, 40–43.

Rang, M. and Wright, J. (1989). What have 30 years of medical progress done for cerebral palsy? *Clinical Orthopaedics and Related Research*, **247**, 55–60.

Reddihough, D., Back, T., Burgess, G., Oke, L. and Hudson, I. (1990). Objective test of the quality of motor function of children with cerebral palsy: Preliminary study. *Developmental Medicine and Child Neurology*, **32**, 902–909.

Reynell, J. K. (1985). *Reynell Developmental Language Scales (Revised)*. NFER–Nelson: Windsor.

Robinson, C. C., Rosenberg, S. A. and Beckman, P. J. (1988). Parent involvement in early childhood special education. In: J. B. Jordan, P. L. Hutinger, J. J. Gallagher and M. B. Karnes (Eds). *Early Childhood Special Education: Birth to Three*. Reston: Council for Exceptional Children, 110–127.

Rose, J., Gamble, J. G., Burgos, A., Medeiros, J. and Haskell, W. L. (1990). Energy expenditure index of walking for normal children and for children with cerebral palsy. *Developmental Medicine and Child Neurology*, **32**, 333–340.

Rosenbaum, P. L., Cadman, D. T., Russell, D. and Gowland, K. (1985). Measurement of motor function in cerebral palsy: issues and problems. *Developmental Medicine and Child Neurology*, **27**, 98–99.

Rosenberg, S. A. and Robinson, C. C. (1988). Interactions of parents with their young handicapped children. In: S. L. Odom and M. B. Karnes (Eds). *Early Intervention for Infants and Children with Handicaps*. Baltimore: Brooks, 159–177.

Schouman-Claeys, E., Picard, A., Lalande, G., Kalifa, G., Lacert, P., Brentanos, E. and Frija, G. (1989). Contribution of computed tomography in the aetiology and prognosis of cerebral palsy in children. *The British Journal of Radiology*, **62**, 248–252.

Shields, J. R. and Schifrin, B. S. (1988). Perinatal antecedents of cerebral palsy. *Obstetrics and Gynecology*, **71**, 899–905.

Sparling, J. (1988). Controlled trials of physical therapy. *Developmental Medicine and Child Neurology*, **30**, 829–830.

Sparrow, S. S., Balla, D. A. and Cicchetti, D. V. (1985). *Vineland Adaptive Behavior Scales*. American Guidance Service: Circle Pines.

Stanley, F. J. (1987). The changing face of cerebral palsy? *Developmental Medicine and Child Neurology*, **29**, 263–265.

Stanley, F. J. and English, D. R. (1986). Prevalence of and risk factors for cerebral palsy in a total population cohort of low-birth weight (<2000G) infants. *Developmental Medicine and Child Neurology*, **28**, 559–568.

Sutton, A. (1984). Conductive education in the Midlands, Summer 1982: progress and problems in the importation of an education method. *Educational Studies*, **10**, 121–130.

Sutton, A. (1987). Evaluating conductive education in children and adults. Presented at summer meeting of the *Society for Research in Rehabilitation*, Newcastle-upon-Tyne.

Szekely, F. (1975). Didactics in conductive pedagogy. In: K. Akos (Ed). *Scientific Studies on Conductive Pedagogy*. Institute of Conductive Education of the Motor Disabled: Budapest, 18–23.

Tardieu, C., Lespargot, A., Tarbary, C. and Bret, M. D. (1988). For how long must the soleus muscle be stretched each day to prevent contracture? *Developmental Medicine and Child Neurology*, **30**, 3–10.

Torfs, C. P., Van Den Berg, B. J., Oechsli, F. W. and Cummins, S. (1990). Prenatal and perinatal factors in the etiology of cerebral palsy. *The Journal of Paediatrics*, **116**, 615–619.

Udwin, O. and Yule, W. (1990). Augmentative communication systems taught to cerebral palsied children—a longitudinal study. 1. The acquisition of signs and symbols, and syntatic aspects of their use over time. *British Journal of Disorders of Communication*, **25**, 295–310.

Vaughan, C. L., Berman, B., and Peacock, W. J. (1991). Cerebral palsy and rhizotomy—a three year follow-up evaluation with gait analysis. *Journal of Neurosurgery*, **74**, 178–184.

Walsh, E. G., Wright, G. W., Brown, K. and Bell, E. (1990). Biodynamics of the ankle in spastic children—effect of chronic stretching of the calf musculature. *Experimental Physiology*, **75**, 423–425.

Watt, J. M., Robertson, C. M. T. and Grace, M. G. A. (1989). Early prognosis for ambulation of neonatal intensive care survivors with cerebral palsy. *Developmental Medicine and Child Neurology*, **31**, 766–773.

Wedell, K. (1960). The visual perception of cerebral palsied children. *Child Psychology and Psychiatry*, **1**, 215–227.

Whitlock, J. A. (1990). Neurophysiology of spasticity. In: M. B. Glenn and J. Whyte (Eds). *The Practical Management of Spasticity in Children and Adults*. Lea and Febiger: London, 8–33.

Whyte, J. and Morrissey, J. (1990). Motor learning and relearning. In: M. B. Glenn and J. Whyte (Eds). *The Practical Management of Spasticity in Children and Adults*. Lea and Febiger: London, 44–69.

Whyte, J. and Robinson, K. M. (1990). Pharmacologic management. In: M. B. Glenn and J. Whyte (Eds). *The Practical Management of Spasticity in Children and Adults*. Lea and Febinger: London, 201–226.

Winters, T. F. and Gage, J. R. (1985). Gait patterns in spastic hemiplegia secondary to cerebral palsy. *Developmental and Child Neurology*, **27**, 105–106.

Woodhill, R. (1991). The Truscott Street Support Unit: pilot programme using the principles of conductive education. *NSW Journal of Special Education*, **14**, 27–30.

Yokochi, K., Horie, M., Inukai, K., Kito, H., Shinabukuro, S. and Kodama, K. (1989). Computed tomographic findings in children with spastic diplegia: correlation with the severity of their motor abnormality. *Brain and Development*, **11**, 236–240.